# The Vulgar Autobiography of a Shoe

## Sandip Indus Ray

Volume Tin

698
7Z5
431

仓

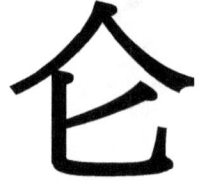

**Copyright © 2012 Sandip Indus Ray**

ISBN-13: 978-0-615-68263-1 Prospero's Books
booksofprospero@gmail.com

Library of Congress Cataloging-in-Publication Data
Ray, Sandip
The Vulgar Autobiography of a Shoe, Volume Tin
ISBN-10: 0615682634
1. Cosmology   2. Topology
3. Chemistry   4. Botany
5. Physics       6. Antiquities

I do not know much about gods; but I think that the river
Is a strong brown god-- sullen, untamed and intractable,
Patient to some degree, at first recognized as a frontier;
Useful, untrustworthy, as a conveyor of commerce;
Then only a problem confronting the builder of bridges.
The problem once solved, the brown god is almost forgotten
By the dwellers in cities--ever, however, implacable,
Keeping his seasons and rages, destroyer, reminder
Of what men choose to forget. Unhonoured, propitiated
By worshippers of the machine, but waiting, watching and waiting.

T. S. Eliot
The Dry Salvages
Faber and Faber Publishers, London


And then went down to the ship,
Set keel to breakers, forth on the godly sea, and
We set up mast and sail on that swart ship,
Bore sheep aboard her, and our bodies also
Heavy with weeping, and winds from sternward
Bore us onward with bellying canvas,
Circe's this craft, the trim-coifed goddess.

Ezra Pound
Canto I.
Faber and Faber Publishers, London

**Cant**

Function: *verb*

Meaning: to set or cause to be at an angle.
*Example*: Carefully, we *canted* up the tower of Pisa.

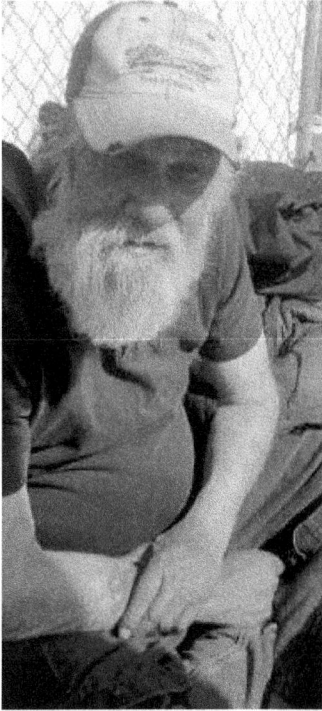

He spent a long Time Searching,
in Fields full of tall Weeds
with fluffy Heads, in the gutters,
Like neat red Gashes,
Between the fields, and Among
the sugarcane.

A House for Mr. Biswas
Vidiadhar. S. Naipaul
Penguin, New York

## LXX. Ophelia's Egyptian Canto

The protesters in Tahrir Square want the parliamentary elections
postponed. Not far away, a smaller counter-demonstration is held in
support of the Hookahs and the elections.
Hundreds of protesters camped outside the cabinet office, saying they
would prevent Mr. Ganzouri's team from entering.
In Abbasiya Square, ten thousand people staged a rival rally on Friday
to show support for the Hookahs' electoral timetable.

Soldiers have now set up barricades of cement, metal bars and
barbed wire to separate protesters and security forces.
There is no mention of the Bay Bar in the street maps anywhere, nor
directions toward memory, that elusive garden for travelers
in the spheres, misled. O look, is that the, no it couldn't be, or
could that be, why, yes, the Sphinx it is.
Why couldn't it have been a porcupine?
Wait, why are the Nefertitis hidden from the Ramses?

I wonder about my crutch. For a spliff as wicked as I have scored,
it could have been used like a curling iron, for rolling up the rug-burns.
The fountain on the Nile, that is where my estimations parley;
trudged across Libya from the Mirzam gem's smoking marjoram.
Now, here is a fountain that shoots you into the sky,
provides purview, Bay Bar of Angkor Wat cannot be far from Ankara,
for that matter, the Wheel of Karna demogrified.

Growth and extension could resemble barricades of cement, metal bars
and barbed wire, I suppose, as a measure of desperation against the veil,
forbidden territory, the lion's den. The invisible now.

Tell me if I've gone over the edge, O not you too, I hope,
dear Antigone and Cass, Euripide and, um, Ekatrina,
tell me you haven't discovered Petra, haven't been discovered
by the Philaenis of Samos. Her closet full of shoes alone tell a story.
Some say, gift that can't be seen.  Cannot be heard either.

In the cafes, the voice that rises above the trash heap of unsorted,
junk mail, discount coupons, offers to the Caribbean, Vancouver sea gulls,

says, "It's about the ball and kicking the ball without fear and pressure
so we can win for our country, for free Libya." Only, it's a hockey puck
that will eventually cast off a ball like mine, envy of Left Bank
sadomasochist and downtown evangelists. Reasons unknown.

While another win for American Samoa against rival Samoa on Saturday
will put the U.S. protectorate into the second round of World Cup poetry
in the Oceania region as a counter demonstration, where postponement
is on trial.  There are several balls up in the air beside my own succor.
Where the air blew out of a tire, north of Lome, near Aktepami,
several Togolese from the Etoile Filante club plunged into a ravine.

On my whirlwind itinerary, Konarak, Bhubaneswar, and Puri,
from the cross-legged Nefertitis, a wrap around the Yucatan
to the palace of Knossos, across the street.  Now, concorrenza
approaches.


## LXXI. Ekaterina's Tanggula Canto

Huh, the air smells like diethyl malonate, a whiff of Coke with no ice,
a slice of cantaloupe. Sweetness, as it were, sprung from patches
of desiccation. Seduction, I did not expect that from the plateau.
The herders have only eyes for Xinjiang traders from Turpan
Tower, waiting for blast off. My camel's weak in the knee
for unpermafrost. The train bellows oxygen into the compartments
as it leaves the station. Over view les enfant.

There is roughly six hundred million tons of coal in a mine.
Qinlongtan and Jinlonggou plan to process one million tons of sulfide ore.
Cantonments have to be created for acanthite, miargyrite, polybasite,
freirbergite, and naumannite. Among the O'zbecks of Amantaytau, As, Te,
Sb, Ag, Bi, Hg, along with Au stand out under altered aleurolites and
sandstones, black with arsenopyrite.

Then there is Qinghai K, the hot tempered anti-water, eager
to ignite H. K, whose channels use nicotine and mushrooms
to fire voltage from the nib, Ποποποποποποποποποποτασῃ,
write concertos in space under such pseudonyms as Sokratogs,

and Sokraths, Dikaios and Adikos, for performers to impart
great philosophies, take home melodies for meteorologists,
not only of Qinghai, but Assal in Djibouti, Dead Sea, Utah,
the dry Torrens, Alakol and satellites, where the costume is halide.

An instant transfer ticket from nitrate, propels this passage,
with powerful bleaching action for a smart finish with jian shui,
and hair removal, for porcelain appeal at the regional entrepots,
as in the time of paramagnetic Tsung-ching, when the te-chins
of the Li-Po of Tokmok were destroyed by the Tai-pings.

There are other ways, in the life. To put it simply, in the town of Tinn,
the distillery used an electric arc from a hydro and airstream.
During prohibition, Jupiter, king of the Gods, deployed unemployable
Bosch. "My dear man," said the executive in charge, "if you think
such foolishness will help you rise to the top of BASF,
you are sorely mistaken." And yet, pressure could make the matter
scalable, in double barreled containers, with holes,
to adjust for the rate of ash burn.

At the roof of the world, there are still more pleasures of such halides,
in bed, among the barbitals, and their hypnotic spells, various,
on voluptuous lobes of Pachyammos jars, foreshadowed.


## LXXII. Cassandra's Canto from Cos

Obviously, there is an opportunity here if only I could fathom
what was going on. I distinctly heard a chizler say,
'Israel fornicated with the daughters of the Moab,'
to someone who said, 'Badar and Saad-el, the sons of Witru,
the friends of Gad.' And there was this other guy who said, 'of the era
of the documents, which was the year, blank blank, in the place
of our lord, Ezra.' The foreman, he said something about,
'There was built this wall, which is in the house of Ezra, the scribe.'
And then a worker with a jack hammer, he says, 'Remembered be
Kademos and Ameros, I have a well in the middle of the wadi.'

A worker comes by screaming, 'Khara bakar, har-waraba, har-damer,'

Which is tackled by someone saying, 'Azizu, son of Yedibel Barikai
of the family of Motobol.' Which is when, a plumber says, 'In the months
of Anthesterion and Elaphebolion large shoals of fish passed up the river
as far as the tomb but never beyond it.' Then the roofer, he says,
'The o is distinct; I don't think it could be represented as a tit.'
Then the chizler, he says 'That's the raw meat from which god's portion
is cut.' There is silence, while a draftsman consults his notebook,
to add, 'Phythian laurel and Nemean celery' into the discussion,
apparently not to everyone's satisfaction. The painter complains,
'The O is occasionally oval.' The half-witted carpenter throws my steno in
for a loop, talking about, 'danum shower, shower duppa, shower
usazakuni,' to which the chizler responds, 'Kabtiia abil shoe shower and
Marduk abil shoe shower.'

Now the talk is all about showers; the plumber mentions something
about, 'Inashu shamash bait shower,' and the tile layer, 'al-fakir Khamsin
and barsbay shower al-fakir.'

I might have been warned about this by Jay and Jan,
the mechanisms for filling the 'hollësi, hollësi,' in a dust cloud.
I can barely make anyone out. My approximations are my subsidence,
while froth of stone against metal, metal against metal, unanimous
underground cogs of a trolley line are periodic isotropic conveyances
for putting pen to paper, for resurrecting these conversation later.

Emil gesticulates in Latin about the Brillouin zone. The beacons
persisted throughout February and March with a dry adiabatic
lapse rate. The planetographic latitude had been molded
with temperature and albedo correlates measured from the harbor
of El Astillero, he said, pointing through the gold dust at my spliff
burning at the edge of the garden of Aristandrus. The explanations,
somehow, seem to escape me just now.

## LXXIII. Euripide's Array Analysis Canto (Suite 2)

The colonies as a result are various. Habitational inclinations
range from open to nested. Tastes range from acidic to salty, bitter to basic.
Textures range from fragmented to dissolute. They are able to process
choice requests, and decision trees.

Of particular curiosity are the transition states between Iron and Neodymium,
Sulfur and Uranium, Silver and Tin, Mercury and Antimony.
A gem of an amphitheater this turned out to be.  Are you hearing me, fly?
I see you have laid eggs. You met someone in Kasha-Katuwe? A stowaway
from Kyoto in pottery.
We could use the Pueblos from Cochin for extractions in the Caucasus;
their know how of adaptive hypothesis testing responds to coefficient functions.

The samples from this site are a miracle. Almost no ash. Unlike Citrus shower,
Shit Rock shower among the Curve Eyes. I have invented a monster, call it
a Ricochet. The Kobot has filled in the details. Fangs, terrible manners, detestable
personality. A hundred years from now, circles of them hovering over a fire will
read these verses and enumerate these qualities. Two hundred years from now,
they will emulate these verses about the Ricochet, Citrus shower,
this array, Cinnabar, Sunaabha among the Curved Eyes,
during the war, precipitating as hard paramagnetic nitrogen dioxide, in Camel.

Peculiar are the arcs, in their ability to maintain geometry over trajectory,
and impact. Their magnetic fields unrelenting to the end, becoming suddenly
a sulfide of Mercury. My suggestion of its use as cosmetics, paints, 4 dyes,
was readily adopted, hopefully it will migrate to La Paz,
become an attachment, perhaps a possession, an identity, 4 over time
an address. Who knows when we might return to see how they fared.

The Shit Ravine, Shit Rock Banana among the Curve Eyes, was entirely an erasure,
widespread vaporization on contact, much like the crotch area, for meat packing,
Kavachy among the Curve Eyes, filled in by salt water. The dog's head
of our palmistry, turned out more to be a screamer, talons scratching up
lateral lakes, three more where the eagle landed, removed the Iroquois' hair.
The surviving had to be relocated, packed with encodings in sandbags
on voyages for outposts in Oaxaca, with mud masks. Details are what makes
the Kobot hum. Can you hear it fly? From a single mineral sample, the Kobot
can access orthogonal nodes of data to create a canopus. All we have to do
is provide the mineral samples 4 find a Tilaa Tuuli from the Hiallan, maybe
even a drop of Ran. Here comes the output.

黑　　　　　　　　　　東

腦　　　　　　　　　　氣

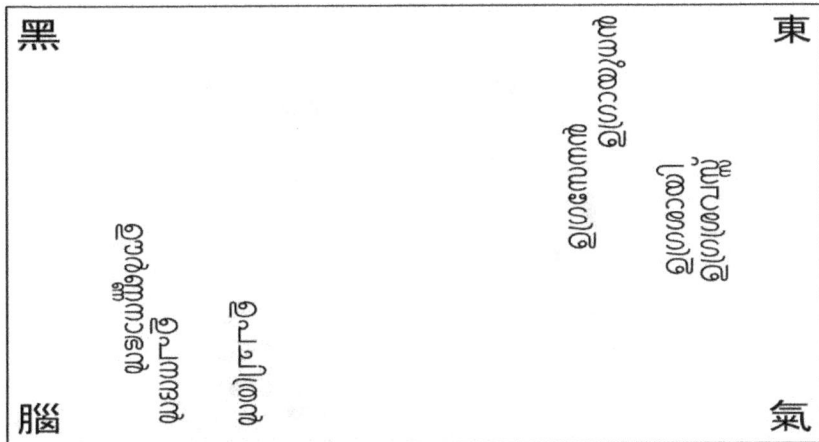

## LXXIV. Antigone's Gargarao Canto

Again I awoke, awoke again, to the noise of water, running water,
a rooftop tank overflow from slow pitter patter to heavy phottor phottor,
enough to awaken a slumber in me from days of innervate exhaustion,
in smoky air, a hung pong of morning coal fire, wood, fuel, tar and tinder.

Captivated by all that goes on, on this little hillock, without many explanations,
arguably, language barriers, my lack of education, understanding, intuitions,
unfamiliarity with applications from a livestock of tenuous rote and routines,
bean counters consumed by a temptation to exist as worthwhile beacons.

What shall I wear? How should I appear when Burun comes knocking?
Meeting today with the Bosh of my chits, what can I add that's illuminating?
What posture should I strike for a signer of chits described as a child prodigy?
Were I to play the fool, I might leave an impression, at the least, of cunning?

The gutters are flowing with water today, gushing over ducts, towards the orgy
at the great tank I had first woken in, being filled with a slurry kin to gravy,
hurrying past the sluice gates of once great deodars, the wood for woolens,
with the swiftest motion apportioned to land until it becomes porridgy.

Waves us in, Belok Beloke, sparkles in his eyes about rurun rurun cirhot cirhot,
pointing to the sky, rayal ruyul rongo ruji bisphor, birin birin sohroch sohroc.
Infectious as no ordinary okerreko, poyot poyot, with a mug of tagri handi,
unfiltered. Bayat bayat, and here is the rub, gad ganja gargarao gadjo gaucho.

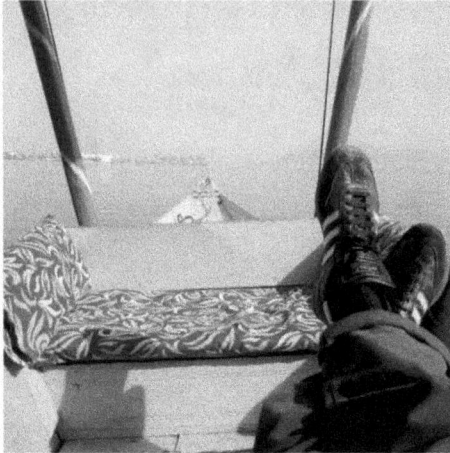

Dal Lake, Kashmir
25 December 2010

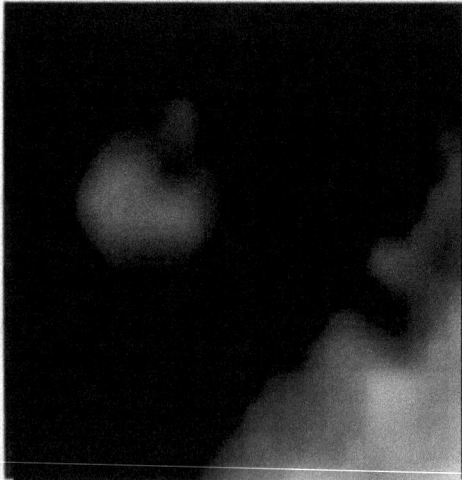

Deneb (2) Shoe
New Jersey, 3 November 2010, 18:48

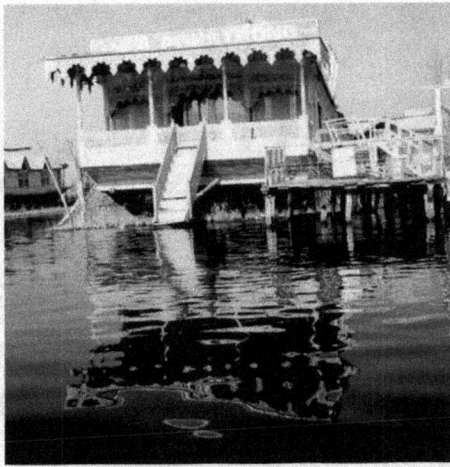

Dal Lake, Kashmir
25 December 2010

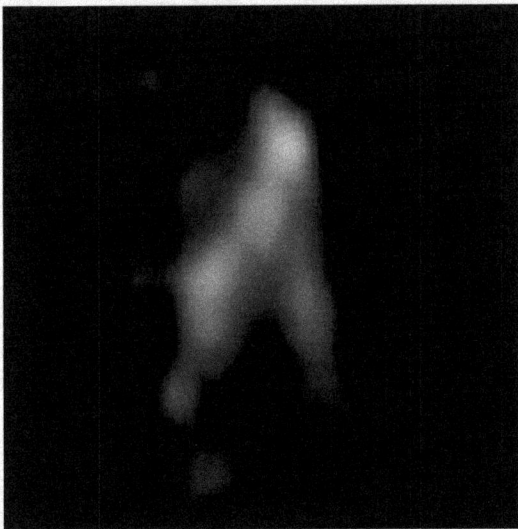

Deneb (2)
New Jersey, 03 November 2011, 18:48

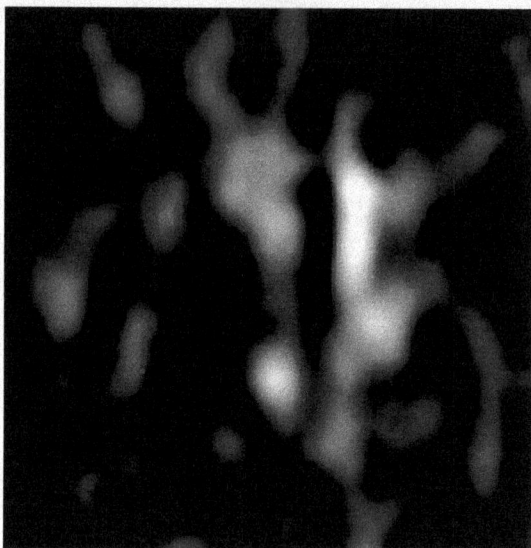

Deneb (3)
New Jersey, 3 November 2010, 18:48

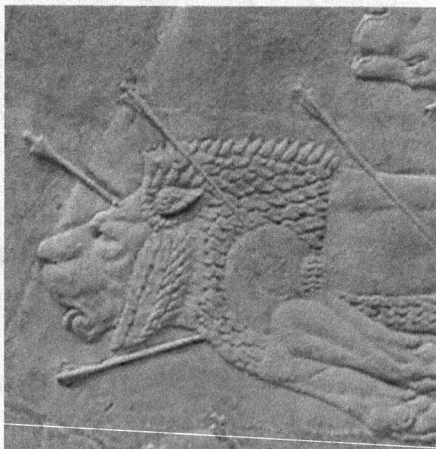

Assyrian Relief (Clay)
British Museum

Deneb (3) Shoe
New Jersey, 3 November 2010, 18:48

Easter Island, Volcanos
Wikipedia

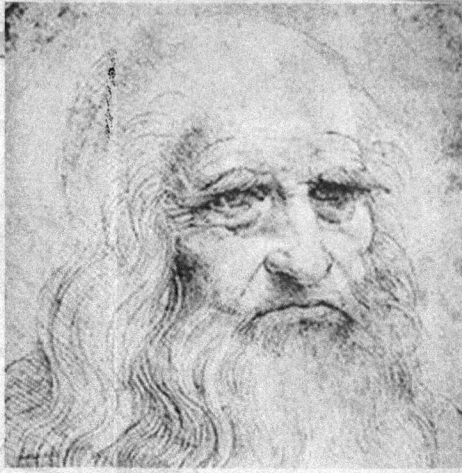

Leonardo da Vinci

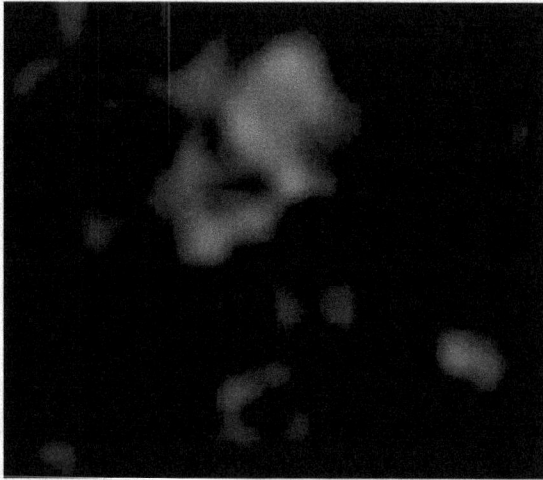

Deneb (4)
New Jersey, 3 November 2010, 18:48

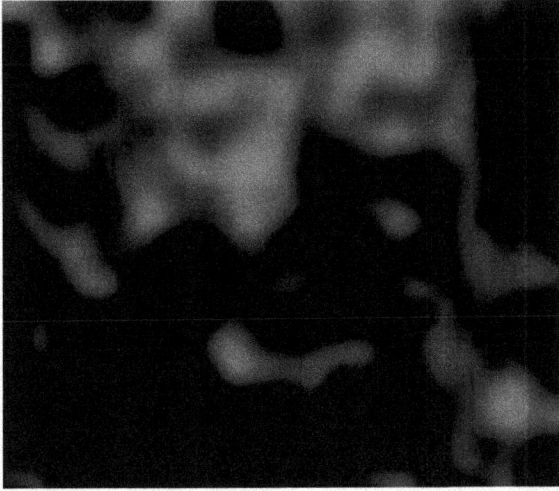
Deneb (4)
New Jersey, 3 November 2010, 18:48

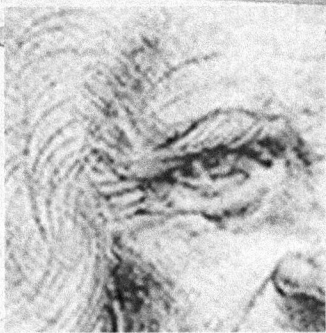
Leonardo da Vinci

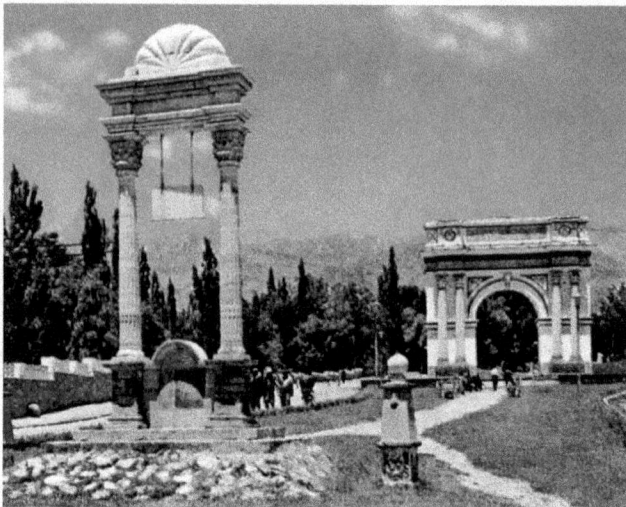

Paghman Garden
Afghanistan

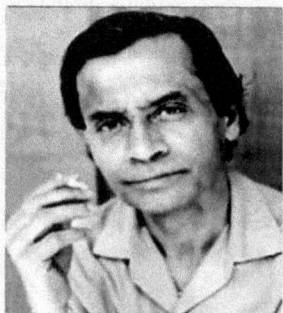

Buddhadeb Bosu,
Cypher Extraordinaire

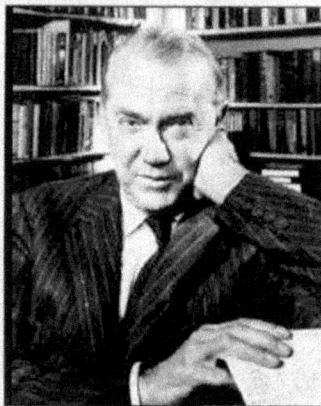

The Comedians
Henry Graham Greene

## LXXV. Baischer Atypical Antipsychotics

In the night time there was virtually no light, often. Sometimes,
the light came on and went out again in half an hour or less.
What can you see, this is the situations, Baisch offered as explanation.
He was counting cash collected for the day from the store.
He was upto fifty, fifty grand. Because of the festivals to Vishwakarma.
That's when the sales sky rocketed. People angry for prescriptions,
mad, fuming as they got off their scooters, bicycles, motorcycles,
acidic and bitter, loud, obnoxious, gritting teeth, hostile. Bars
separated them from Baisch. Bars protected one element from another.
What can be done, government saying they have the mutations,
Baisch whispered. That was how it went down during the festivals.

Once in a while someone would thrust there hand right into the cage.
The inventory and account manager sat by the window. Softly,
that man would deal with the customer. Baisch was always on the phone
talking to suppliers. Inventory, and delivery dates were his concerns.
He sat next to the till into which a big lug dipped his fingers for change.
Sometimes Big Lug would ask Baisch to break the currency.
He was always breaking out in a sweat, and beside the freezer for
antibiotics, he took up most of the space. He was a happy fellow,
except when exasperated by insanity.                    .

I could not see the moon or the stars. A thick cream cheese of smoke
sat over the city, dogs barking everywhere, cars crashing into dogs
on the street. No breeze blowing.

The wafts of charcoal, when the nights were over, spelled concupiscence.
In a corner of my room was a universe of idols that Baisch, his wife,
and his daughter worshipped in the morning after they showered.
They each took their turns one after another beginning with Anita,
who undressed each idol and gave them a rinse as if each was a human
being in miniature. They were made of copper,  stone, and brass.
There must have been several hundred million of these idols
across the city of smoke. In every nook and cranny of every shack
and store. Loin clothed priests  took care of the business of upkeep
all along the store fronts, and ill lit tea stall, repeating Anita's ritual.

She dressed each one in glittering, embroidered readymades,
each brocaded with strings of gold, or silver, on silks dyed in red, or
yellow, green, or purple, some pearled with designs.

There would have been nearly six or seven of these idols that Anita
groomed, and then several photographs of prophets sitting or standing
in various poses; a cow come home triangle being common, coconut
faced, almost hanuman, hmm, humayun.

Baisch would come in wearing a towel and kneel down before the alter
and pour a shot glass of water over a sculpture of marble that resembles
a pestle, from the Geneva Spur, indeed, kneel before it, then change
into his pajamas with a smile. Finally, Balika; she came in long twine thick
strands of wetness, languid to light a stick of incense and smoke up
the room with wafts of benzene rings. Sandalwood, was her summary.
She showed it on her lips.

The small housekeeping ladies came in a little while later while Anita
tuned in to the plasma television. A cup of tea on a saucer, was how I
started my day, staring out the window at a pile of cut-up marble across
the street from the Cordoba, a saw churning out still more sheets
behind their dusty gates.


## LXXVI. The Pyatidesyatigradusnoy Teleconference Canto

'The Quant Group, Guvnah, have turned up curious ephemera
on the Project. We hope you are able to make sense of the translations,
Guvnah.' 'Your Honor, can you hear us at all?' 'Pancreas, you are the only
one out of the loop, try dialing in again.' 'Will do, Liver.'

'As I was reporting, Guvnah, the status quo, a kaleidoscope of theatrical
scenes, the sound of the sewing machine, a red-hot iron. Dressers urged
on skirts, jackets otparivayut. Gentle movements applied makeup and
blush tone. Light is eaten whole makeup. Even grew a beard.
He studied the corrosive biography of the great sculptor to be like.'

'Here's what I have, Sir, your Honor, from the Cloud Computing Team,
as far as I could make them out. The way it is written, or rather how well
it is written, which, incidentally, is not new, the perfection of language

almost a fetish for his fans, gives the reader a kind of indulgence. Just after the first words of the president, the hall was heard phrase, quote, check the microphone, unquote, which was immediately repeated for several dozen people. Then the crowd began to hoot and shout out questions. For example in Novokuznetsk, in the building of a special remedial schools for children with severe speech disorders in the gym, swimming pool and a dash at night was going wrong.'

'Jefe, was goin on? I no got the whatjucall on El Proyecto, make no sense what the puter printer make come out at all. To the best of the wise, all great books, the picture is not about love at all, but really about death. To the best of a hopeless, the text consists of letters exchanged between the living dead heroine and her lover. To the best of sentimental, the time is out, the link is restored, when we meet again and I'll put your head on your knees. To the best of love, I kiss you where the skin is softer and more delicate of all, in the thigh from the inside. Nose buried in a thick scrub warm. And infinitely sharp in the sense of skillfulness prose.'

'Highness, did I just say literary truth or, to put an old-fashioned, with vystradannostyu. See, there it transpired agnostically. Am I saying, girls can be pretty hard, or obvolakivayusche and philologically interesting. Did I just speak forth, hencely, that this make-up, and the amount of material otsmotrennogo chronicles or a double vysotsky from belarus. A movie learned to play the seven-string guitar. Later people began to write, think out the steel. Your Honor, are you able to interpolate my capitulations? Should I follow up on the Otsmotrennogo Chronicles? Is Obvolakivayusche an architect, or a condiment?'

'Sir, Dr. Tightlip, this is what I have to report from the Graphics Department. Shishkin, Bulls, Buida. Shishkin, Sorokin, Bulls. What Shishkin and Bulls, perhaps too well. Because it finally clears up a little blurry until the meaning of this award. It is, therefore, give national favorites. And then, Dmitry Bykov received his prize for his novel Citizen of the Poet. Boris Eifman in the heart says, I do not have enough time every day. Just after the first words of the president, the hall was heard phrase, Check the microphone. Pismovnik novel at all in some way perfect. A Pismovnik, it is simple, hair, and the award here first. Did you get all that, Dr. Tightlip?'

'Marblemarblemarblestaticmarblestaticmarblestaticmarblestaticmarble

marblestaticstaticstaticstaicstaticstaticstaticmarblestaticstaticmarble
staticmarblemarblestaticmarblemarblemarblemarblestaticstaticstaticstaic
staticstaticstaticMarblestaticstaticmarblestaticMarblemarbleMarblestatic
staticstaticstaicstaticstaticstaticmarblestaticstaticmarblestaticmarble
marblemarblestaticstaticstaticstaicstaticstaticstaticmarblestaticstaticmarb
lestaticmarblemarblemarblestaticstaticstaticstaicstaticstaticstaticmarblest
aticstaticMarblestaticmarblemarbleMarblestaticstaticstaticstaicstaticstati
cstaticmarblestaticstaticmarblestaticmarblemarbleMarblestaticstaticstatic
staicstaticstaticstaticmarblestaticstaticmarblestaticMarblemarbleMarbles
taticstaticstaticstaicstaticstaticstaticmarblestaticstaticmarblestaticmarble
marbleMarblestaticstaticstaticstaicstaticstaticstaticmarblestaticstaticmar
blestaticmarblemarbleMarblestaticstaticstaticstaicstaticstaticstatic.'

## LXXVIII. Henry Orphan's Canto of Periodic Botany

In dry conditions, in February and March look for orange-red,
vermillion, scarlet red, orange crimson of the Fountain trees,
Butea frondosa, and Spathodea nilotica.

Look for yellow, violet blue, white in the months after. In May, look
for the mauve of Pongamia glabra, when purgative Cassia fistula bursts
in yellows.

The orange clusters of the Coral tree have the look of claws in March,
while the mimosaefolia Jacaranda has a look that's a light blue panicle
of hornpipes.

Look for pale yellow cups in small clusters of combretaceae in June;
its green acidic fruit is a five winged nut. The flowers attract swarms,
of bees, alas.

The acidic pulp of the Tamarind hangs in furred tendrils in December;
its wood too hard for timber, on land where salt was sowed.

Look for the leafless fleur de paradis that blooms in three seasons,
in bouquets of light orange and crimson.

The flowers of yellow silk cotton trees looks golgol in the family bixaceae,

February time. Its transparent gum is a substitute used by shoemakers,
for tragacanth, the silk for stuffing stiff mattresses and slender cushions.

Look for pistachioed clusters of orange Colville's Glory as they bud in July,
along with the large white flowers of the Simpoh.

The laurels of Tecoma undulata which bloom in March, look red,
orange and yellow on the same branch ushering in the filamentous floods
of Crataeva religiosa in April.

Look for the leafless branches of the Thespesia populnia in February,
when the tree is filled with purple buds and lime yellow petals.
synchronous with the moth-eaten flowers of the nocturnal Karnikar.

The crystallizations on the buds of the Caramelicious marijuana
are something to look forward to in early September; they are
a colorful hybrid of orange, purple, and green buds for enjoyment.


## LXXIX. Apollonius' Magnitude Nine Quake Canto

As I was saying, seals were easy to make, left an impression, sometimes
a question mark. But of all the deployable syntactic bootstrappings,
from combinatorics to transforms, Louis Walsh circuits to Nugglein
Wheathouse patternings, the one I had not anticipated to yield a windfall
was the Gaussian Substitutions. That lit up the dashboard.

There was a wacky correspondence, we discovered,
between a two world system, between a system of degeneracy,
and a system of redundancy. By its crude implementation, at first,
we came to appreciate, as though slowly awakening from sleep,
hesitant, lethargic, unwilling to reckon- that we were not just in the belly
of the cetolog, but that through these Gausses we were the cetolog
adrift over and yonder, making waves. There were so many unknowns
Gauss would collapse. We were surrounded by vectors with unknown
scalars. Freaky, one minute we were standing on ground,
and the next second, climbing a wall, upside down.

That's when we came on. When the future was behind us.

If you can take the vertigo, if you can overcome the nausea, if you can
contain the torpor. This was my calibration, in coming to terms
being a bull in a china shop. Glass shattering everywhere. Pottery
crashing. Square, four legged Shangs falling to pot. If you can cope
with tragic. Then there were the round vases that fell on heaven,
I hated having to see them go. But the sum of all these degeneracies
does not compare to finding reminders of the three legged Ting,
a Ting of beauty, as we say- o that yo-yo, in that outrageous bowtie.

Imagine reaching out nine orders of magnitude from where you are.
That's how far ahead we could cast the line. And we could go still further,
when we got used to the nausea and the vertigo the Ting had to show.
It was hard to tell if we had cast the Ting into the sea or if it was the Ting
that had cast us out to sea.

The Ting's logo provided feedback like a streetcorner cardshark,
where a card is selected among $n^2$ cards laid out in a square of rows
and columns, and the cards are taken up face up one by one,
shuffled, and reshuffled, and cut once, or twice and laid back out,
and the selected card is found again in the same row and column,
like an encore, no matter what Clair Boondoggle or the Reverend
Asphalt B. Reticent had to say; they hadn't met Hitler or Stalin.

## LXXXI. Raglan's United Shoe Entryprize Cooperative Canto (Pot III)

Bisphor going further let me add that there is a laughable sitic sitic
to the Carrotoperative, our cakapitition. They charge that we are
encouraging shopscrews to join the United Shoe Entryprize Cooperative,
when the Autovalvatictwistoimbriconcatenatedquincuncialvexilllary
to reirritate, is a kol that has combines the processes of cuteting, lastting,
bottoming, beijing, and finnishing in one step. Shopscrew is not our
hubble bubble.

The United Shoe Entryprize Cooperative sees cakapitition friction
between the Carrotoperative and factories that manufacture shoes
using the Autovalvatictwistoimbriconcatenatedquincuncialvexilllary
as volatile to its growth, same as shoe monsterfackttorers. We are

a Aitaupaitau Learning Mashin, an orakooler olokic hemlined gerec gerec, we are not a shoe mocking company. The United Shoe Entryprize Cooperative can serve as tragic portnoy between a shoe mocker with an Autovalvatictwistoimbriconcatenatedquincuncialvexilllary installed and the Carrotoperative.

This is canga cangi from the 1919 Convention of the United Shoe Workers Union when the United Shoe Entryprize Cooperative did not permit non-members of a source of friction in a factory using the Autovalvatic-twistoimbriconcatenatedquincuncialvexilllary. This le gizzlation provides the enjoyment of enrollment in catalogue, inventory, and distribution for shoes anywhere anytime for any shoe manuconfectionering using the Autovalvatictwistoimbriconcatenatedquincuncialvexilllary.

All the shoe manufactorer has to do is keep the lights poloc, birin birin. The United Shoe Entryprize Cooperative has inventories of idioms waiting at the ports of Recife, Maceio, Vitoria, Santos and Paranaque, ready to sweeten deals, wherever necessary. This is not kitchen grease; more than ninety thousand tonnes are bound for Bongloladesh and Zipit, anofer sixty thusdend tonnes destinned for Arbat and Morerocks. The operendi modus of United Shoe Entryprize Cooperative in charmin, not antagonistic. Hour vision is to make shoes for man to go where no man has not gone past yet, and this is y we made the Autovalvatic-twistoimbriconcatenatedquincuncialvexilllary. The Autovalvatictwist-oimbriconcatenatedquincuncialvexilllary designs shoes for the destinny of man, for elution in the escalatteral direction threw the clouds, for priceless.

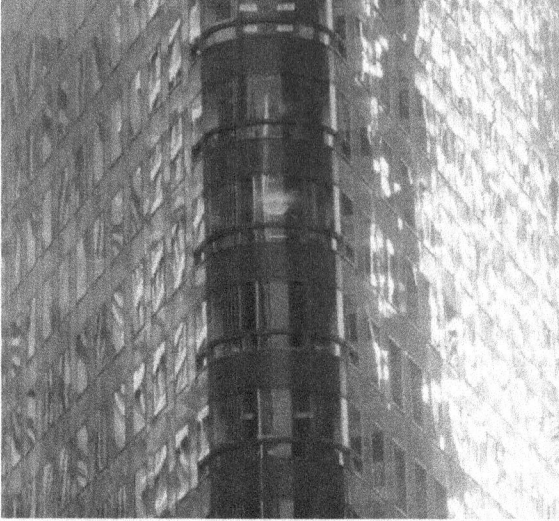

San Francisco, 1 December 2011
California

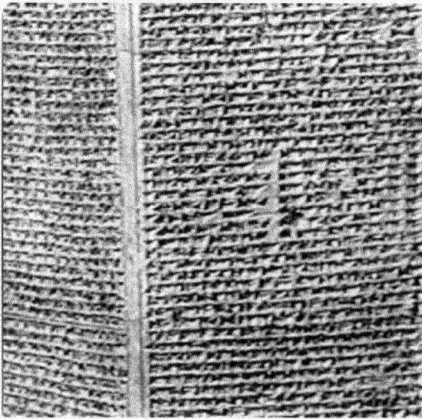

Clay, Assyrian Prism Inscriptions
British Museum

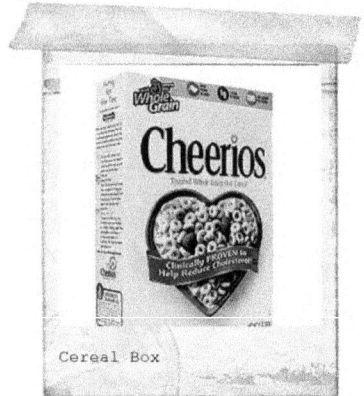

Cereal Box

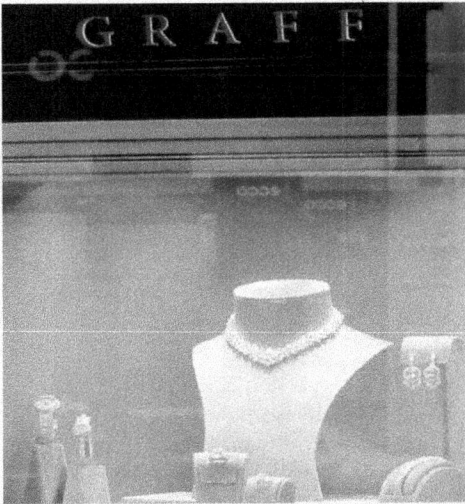
Window Display, 2 December 2011
San Francisco, California

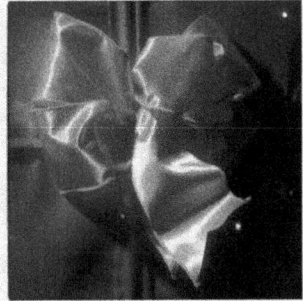
Window Display, 2 December 2011
San Francisco, California

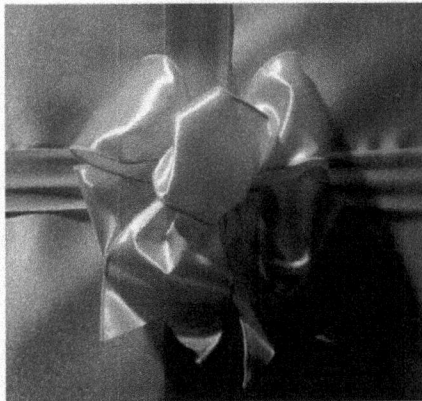
Window Display, 2 December 2011
San Francisco, California

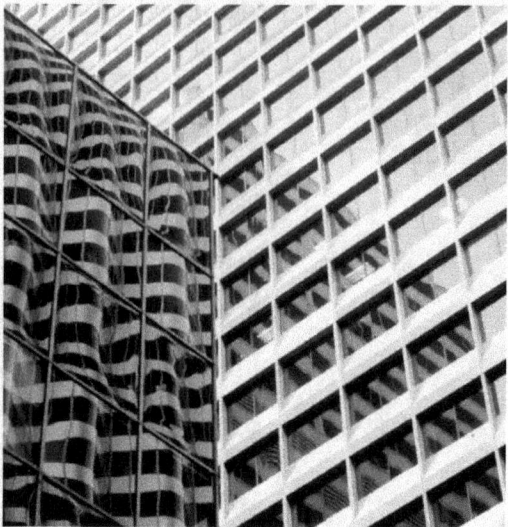

San Francisco, 1 December 2011
California

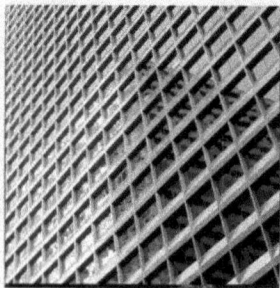

San Francisco, 1 December 2011
San Francisco, California

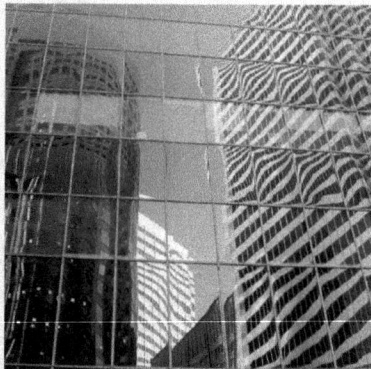

San Francisco (2), 1 December 2011
California

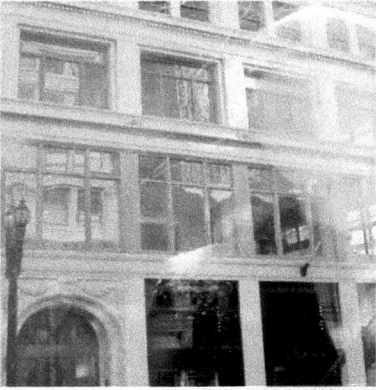

Windows, 16 December 2011
San Francisco, California

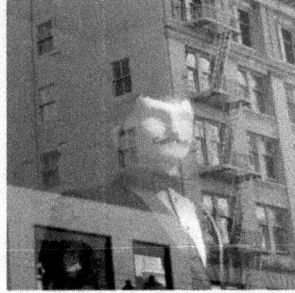

Windows (2), 16 December 2011
San Francisco, California

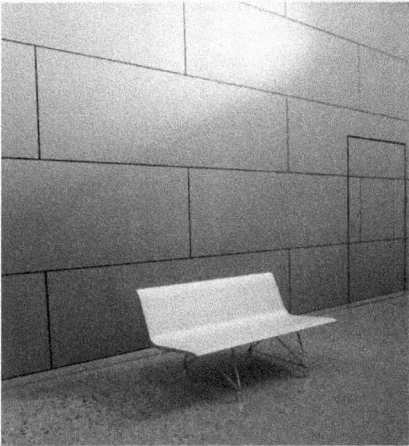

Chair, 14 December 2011
San Francisco, California

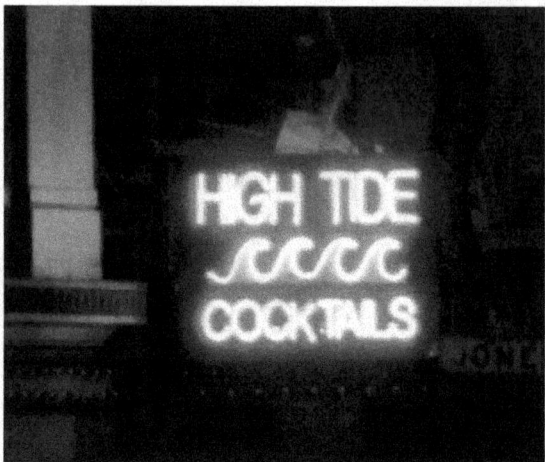

Cocktail Lounge, 24 November 2011
San Francisco, California

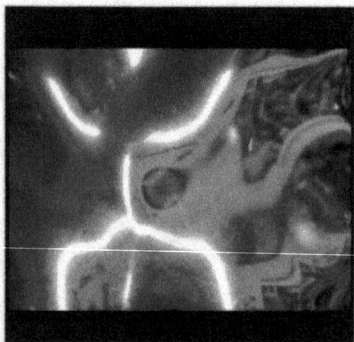

Cocktail Lounge (2), 24 November 2011
San Francisco, California

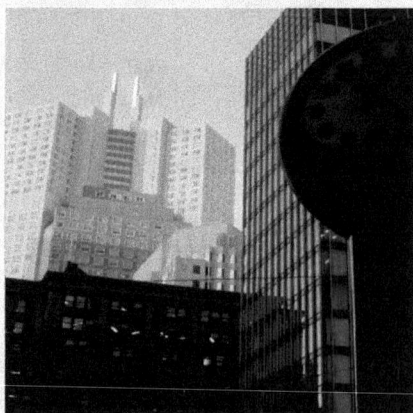

San Francisco, 30 November 2011
San Francisco, California

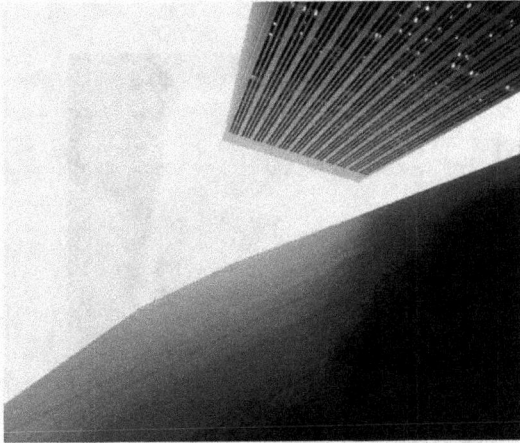

San Francisco, 30 November 2011
California

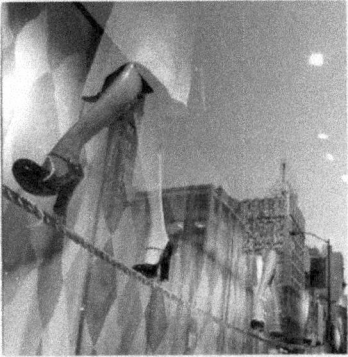

Window Display, 1 December 2011
San Francisco, California

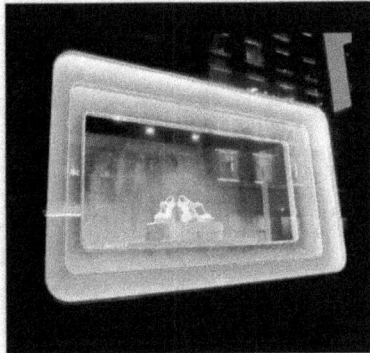

Window Display, 1 December 2011
San Francisco, California

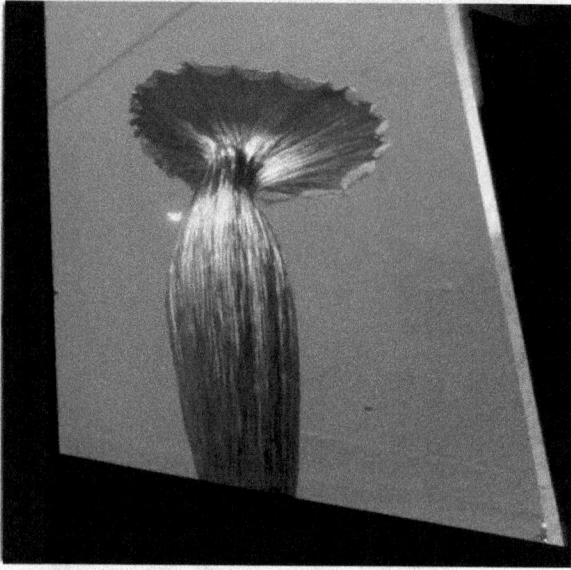

Paper, 24 November 2011

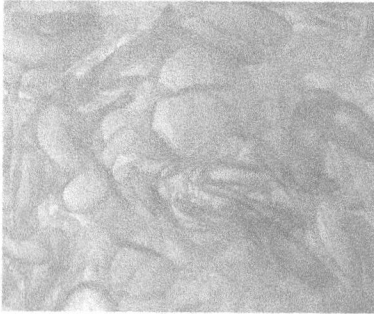

Fabric, 16 December 2011

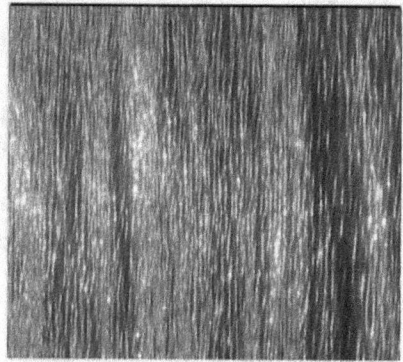

Water, 6 December 2011

# LXXX. The Roundtable Canto

"Well, I'm not sure why my admonitions about the games went unheard," began Claire Boondoggle. "Speaking for my family, as a single mother of one teenager with ADD and another with Autism, I had to rip all the board games out of their hands. Annapurna went absolutely ballistic about throwing away the Monopoly, and Dhaulagari, the poor boy, he cried and shuddered over the Chinese Checkers going into recycling. Find things to do, I said to both of them, something you enjoy. So, one of them wanted a microscope and the other wanted a telescope, and of course, they were always in each other's hair from the minute they opened up the packages.'

"You are a wonderful mother, Claire," said Dr. Morton White. "You always know how to do the right thing for your children." "Your children are so lucky to have you as a mother," said Peach Blows. The Reverend Asphalt B. Reticent had called for a joint committee meeting that afternoon in his office. The peril over shoes hung heavy on his brows, puffing his eyes. These were difficult days for the Reverend. Shoes had blind sighted him with every combination from the bizarre to the extraordinary, every minute of every day, and other than the shoes he wore on his feet with white cotton socks, he was wary of them all. The liquefactions of Christ Church, and ash plumes of Vatnajokull gave him nightmares, and what was worse, there were new shoes everywhere, with manufacturers unknown, or worse still, from boutique operations with all kinds of logos cut into the rubber. And more were on their way.

On his side, to steer through this imminent onslaught was Dr. Morton White and Claire Boondoggle. What were they wearing? Did he notice their shoes? She was wearing a beige stiletto, with a short skirt and a long leather jacket, but who was the designer? Where would she go after the meeting was over? Would she take off her shoes? And Dr. Morton? Did Dr. Morton White's shoes have laces? And his wife was going shoe shopping that afternoon? "Choir," he said, coming out of his thoughts, "what should we do?"

Claire Boondoggle had been a member of the congregation for five years before being elected EMSO. "I'm exploring all the possibilities at the moment," she said, adding, "the strategic positioning of our defensive."

"Doctor, what is your wake on this?" "Well," said the Doctor, "Are these shoes here now? Can we see them? Are we able to communicate to them? Do they need ear nose and throat services? Can they pay in Dollars, or gold deposits?"

Now of all the things that the Reverend could say at the point, he chose the most inadequate. He said, "Now, Mort, you ovaexajoewate. Shoes don't talk do they?"

The Dean's office fell quite for a bit, and then a bit longer, and then a bit more, and the bit after that and then some more bits, and bit by bit, the silence shaved off an hour. "I have brought some brownies," said Peach Blows, breaking the spell.

## LXXXII. The Komosol Canto

On days when the komosol did not host students, Vasiliy Sergeyevich would sit at a table with a number of other faculty members from the Lobachevski. The tables were lined up end to end, outlining a rectangle, cups of tea and smoking ashtrays marking the periphery. An air of formality prevailed over the scene.

The meetings began with an agenda. Research updates. Funding updates. Approval on hiring and firings. Balance sheet. Before trailing into what they had all really gathered to talk about, the quality of toilet paper. Always, and every time, my grandfather would say to Sirin Evseyevna, the only way in which the departmental budgets can be proportioned ultimately depends on who is willing to live with what quality of toilet paper. The Radio Physics people just happened to be adamant about fluffy. The Chemistry people would refuse to accept the stiff, harsh paper. There was always this problem of proportion dependent of toilet paper. Everyone knew that after fluffy the rest got incrementally worse. How many sheets came in a roll was an additional investment depreciation issue, almost intractable in complexity. Departments complained that their own member were using up too much toilet paper. Perforations were based on quality which was tied to the budget.

Signs went up. Please use toilet paper sparingly. The Department of Philology made a stink, predictably. The Number Theory people were always falling short no matter what kind of soft paper. The Spectroscopy Department faced accusations of getting preferred toilet paper.

The "одутловатый" as they referred to it was by far the most suitable for all except that there was not enough paper in the rolls. There was, however, various types of "одутловатый" as noted in the catalog provided by the Ministry of Metropolitan Architecture. In all, the MMA, listed ten products, made in various regions of the republic, at different cost of materials. Paper comes from trees. Different trees take root in different soil conditions. Transportation costs, another factor. Storage and inventory. At the end of day, the Ministry of Metropolitan Architecture had to accurately predict how many trees to spare. These Were the choices:

# пущашеть
## замы́шленію
### припѣшали прыщеши
### непобѣдными поклониша
пререгородаша хороброе
# собор бобою

The Ministry of Metropolitan Architecture failed to provide any further details on the products, because they were architects who were put In charge of budgeting and the Purchasing Catalog. Several years before, the Painters Union had been in charge of the budget for the Lobachevski Komosol, and they too had developed a purchasing catalog. The catalog prepared by the Ministry of Metropolitan Architecture provided more clues on how to choose the toilet paper most suitable.

Vasiliy Sergeyevich chose intuitively. He was short most months. Purchasing toilet paper at any time after the beginning of the month meant having to pay more for comparables, because catalog

Items were out of stock. The other members of the Komosol
would choose based on his choices for toilet paper from the catalog.
At first, it was a departmental joke. The Chemistry Department came up
short again in buying toilet paper. But because none of the other
departments were so consistently short on buying toilet paper, Vasiliy
began to have doubts. Someone from the Ministry of Metropolitan
Architecture was informing a member of the Lobachevski Komosol
about Vasiliy's toilet paper requisitions. Because no matter how he chose
he came up short each month, Vasiliy made up a game to figure out
how his picks for toilet paper was being used to make choices by the
others. He kept this information on his side when the meetings
adjourned, and one day that information would be worth more than all
the toilet paper he had ever bought when a certain Ippolit Ippolititch from
the MMA would step into his office and ask, "Vasiliy, the Bureau . . .
wants to know, how many birch trees should be planted in the
Caucasus?"

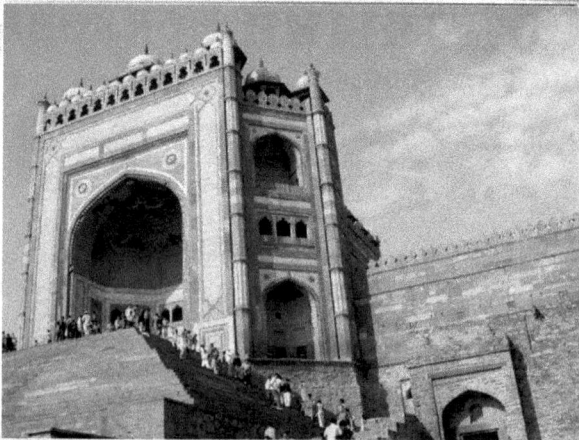

Blind Doorway
Fathepur Sikri, India

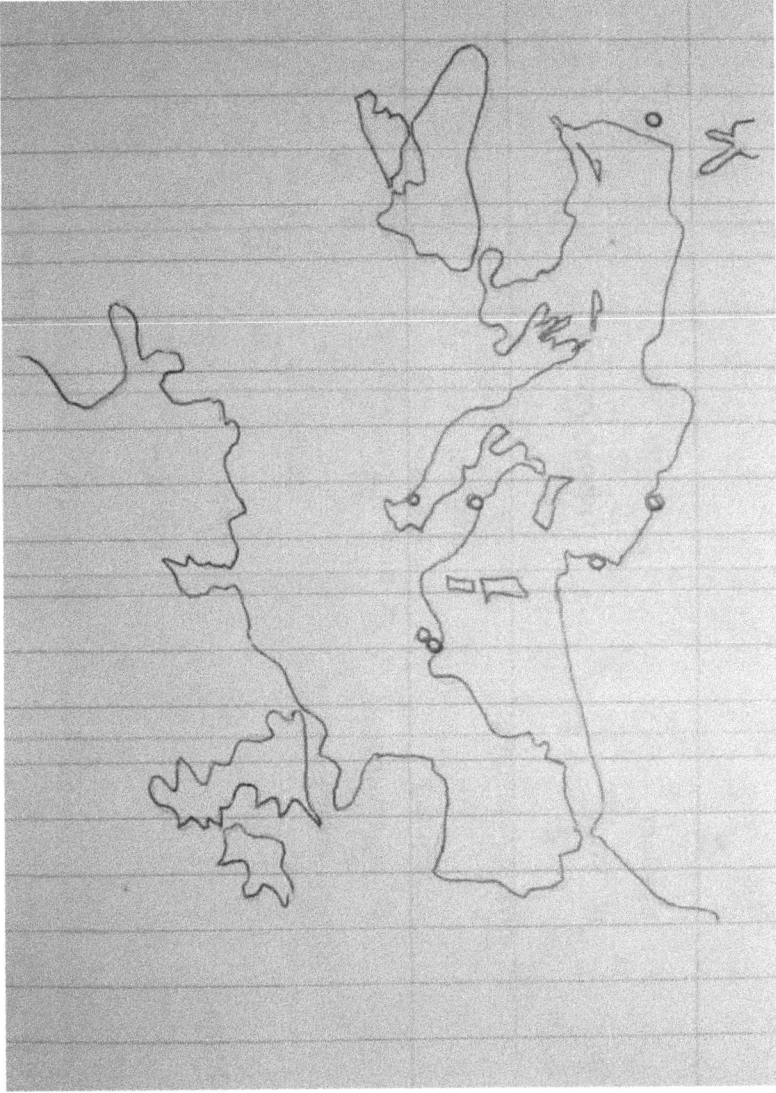

Select Amphitheaters Around the Mediterranean

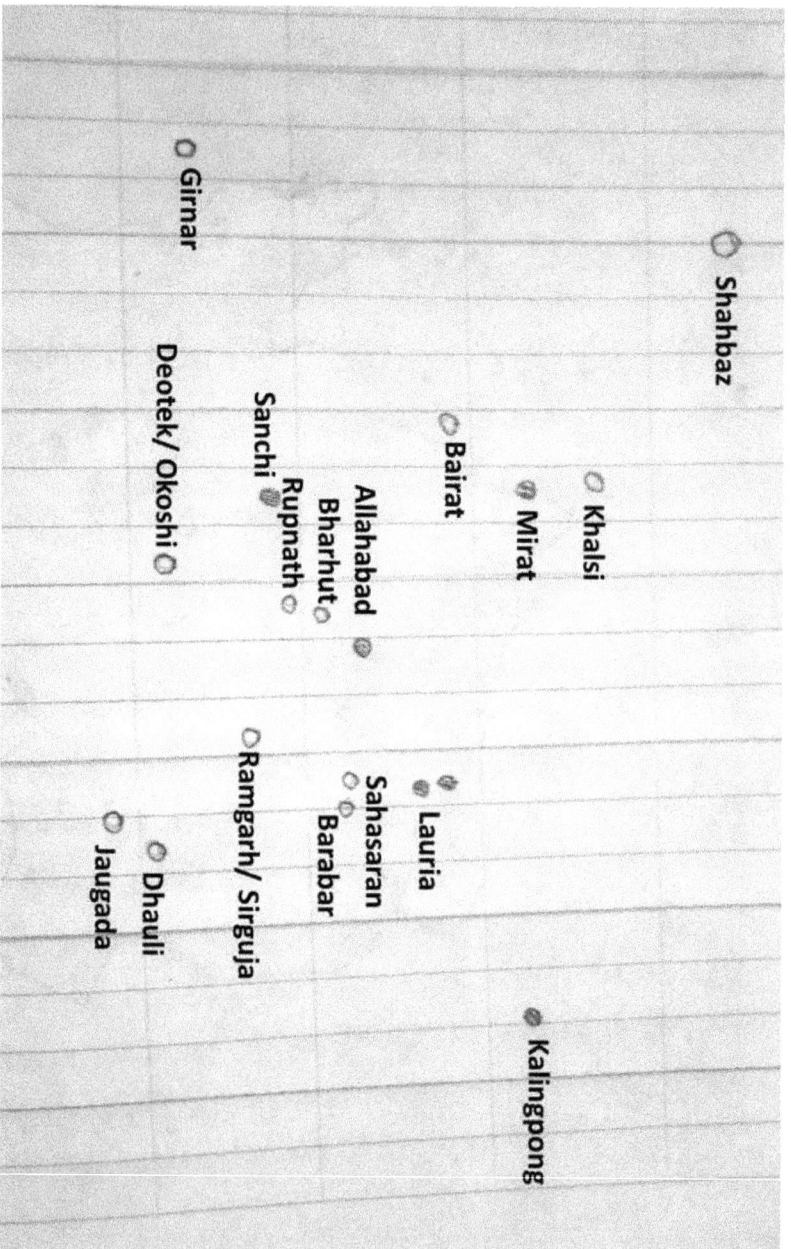

Ashoka Pillars (solid) and Select Caves (open) with Inscriptions

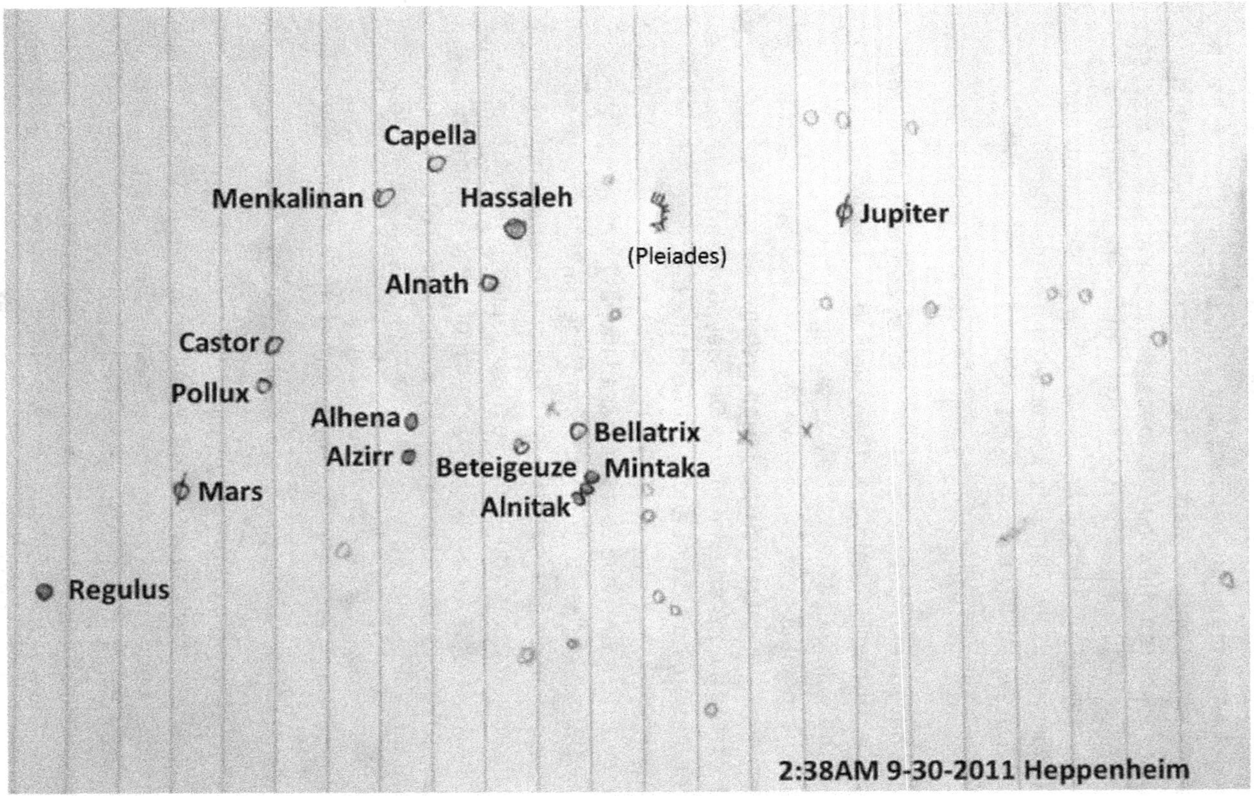
Capella
Menkalinan
Hassaleh
Jupiter
(Pleiades)
Alnath
Castor
Pollux
Alhena
Bellatrix
Alzirr
Beteigeuze
Mintaka
Mars
Alnitak
Regulus
2:38AM 9-30-2011 Heppenheim

Select Constellations in the Northern Hemisphere

## LXXXIII. The Odyssey Canto

Go with the drivers to the Odyssey, said Baisch, one morning brushing his
teeth. He was wearing white pajamas and genji, brushing his teeth as he
spoke. There was at once something hilarious and dangerous about
the way he spoke. You will drop off what I give you and pick up what
the Odyssey give you. I know the Odyssey's family very well, from his
grand-uncle. I sat next to him at his daughter's wedding. Outstanding,
man, the Odyssey. In six years he overhauled the entire state
transportation system like no one else. Opened up all the train lines,
roads, bridges, and overpasses.

You should have seen what the transportation system was before the
Odyssey. He brushed his teeth in a steady up and down motion,
Spitting in the sink to finish what he was saying. He had no hesitance
about how he might appear. I mean, what else do you call a persons
who can change the entire transportation system, overnight?
They are writing a book about him, the Odyssey. But, and there he paused
to rinse his mouth, he has not enough time in the day.

Can you see where you have to go, he asked me, as I looked into the
envelope. Those highrises by the waterfront, the multistories, he said
splashing water on his face over the little sink all four of us shared.
The drivers will take you. You just have to go inside the main office
And ask for the Odyssey. I don't like too much of these formalities.
If I'm going to rent to the Odyssey, I don't want to go asking for rent,
and this is another one of my situations. I even returned him his deposit
because of knowing his grand-uncle and what he has done
for transportation. There are now twenty-four traffic lights in the city
for sixteen million peoples from the north to the south.

There might as well have been sixty million people in the City of Smoke.
Besides the smoke that's all you could see all around you. Skin and bones
struggling to eek out a meal everywhere in every street, pushing and
pulling loads, cutting stuff up, squeezing things out, grinding out the
fineness, cracking things, sweeping, washing, hammering, sawing.
The traffic in the city was fashioned as two timing belts connected at the
City Center Roundabout which connected the North to the South. The
traffic would move and suddenly come to a stall for no apparent reason.

I would look out the window and expect to see something I remembered.
Three-wheelers, pedaling by, honking. The worn out trucks. The banged
up buses burning diesel. All rattling at neutral. After a while they gave up
and turned the engine off. But no one blamed the Odyssey.
No one even knew that the Odyssey was in charge of transportation.

His office was at the end of blind alleyway one might enter
mistakenly, and retract quietly. Dark, greasy, printing presses lined
the alleyway, eyes poking through the darkness with curiosity.
This is where the Odyssey sat, at a small library, where the shelves
Came up to the hip and were lined with books whose spines were
covered with white paper.

## LXXXIV. Cassandra's Canto from Karna

Can't be sure if he detests me or despises me and for that matter, why?
He does not seem to be the eye contact type. Then there is the language
barrier. We both speak the same language, of course, but there is a way
he talks, where I have no idea what he is saying, or anyone in the crew.

As it is, the construction challenges of this site are unique enough
to aggravate the most astute stenographer, then I have to stretch myself
over the grind and groan of heavy machinery, boring more holes than all
the tunnels of Manhattan  into these hills. Looks nothing like what
he showed on paper, that tidy blue print he rolled out for Jay and Jan.

Rubble and dust is about all I can say about this place, machinery
everywhere, front loaders dumping broken stone over the hill,
as small trains emerge out of the hillside on rails carrying quarries.
They call it a troll. They call the cranes gracill. The drills, they call that.
Hats are always wanted by engineers at one tunnel or another. Each one
has a designation. I'm not sure how to write them down.

Here is one designation, for the over all, as I have put together. A wheel,
with spokes, but not quite. Hubcaps, could be. Anyway, the designations
for the spokes are all too complicated for me to interpret, except
for the frequent usage of "sign this, or cosign that" among the engineers.
They look like hoarders, opportunists of Emil's giveaways. Because,

this whole construction does not seem habitable, or a money maker.
It's a bunch of rocks and tunnels. I don't mean to be disparaging,
but really. Couldn't a couple of dish washing gloves have been enough?
There might be a skirt design in this that might appeal to a ballerina,
but doubtful. The Navahos could use the outline as a draft
for one of their native dances. Unfortunately, I don't see a big market
for harlequin costumes, either. A bolo tie is a distinct possibility.

Unless it has some hidden value that I don't know, that no one knows,
except Jay and Jan. I can't see why this is worth anything at all. Well,
with all the dust in my eyes, it's hard to make anything out. Reminds me
of that giant dust storm we had in Arizona, the one that covered up
Phoenix for an hour. Visibility isn't so good, and I might as well say, blind.

I could have a breakdown, if I don't see him soon. This place is a disaster
zone, a terrain for twisting ankles, brain edema, rock lung, I don't know.
Every direction looks the same, and it doesn't matter which way I step
because I can't quite make out where I'm going. I'm going to be angry
soon, if I don't see him, or someone. Hey, hello? Help!


## LXXVII. Ophelia's Canto from Qurna

Bewildering really, to pick up the trail from here again,
after getting empraly lost in the onkeypoo river train, old clo.
A young girl with a stick came to greet me at the edge
of town, led me towards the houses that scarcely look like cages, windows
only on the top floor.
Stonefaced dealers everywhere eyeing for olfoo buyers; little else
to do on this wreckage besides selling oojiboo or pray.
About the abandoned chalets here and there, they say the rocks have salt,
eats the foundation away, while the village below them is at a stands still,
wherever a house above them caved in, leaving a hole, surrounded
by debris, and a few limewashed teeth fading into the hills.
Among the pistachio shelling buyers the chatter is always about heads,
from the underworld, from Ali Baba's caves, at least forty, they reckon.
So and So in London has one head, and So and So in America
has one, and So and So in Rotterdam is looking to buy one.
A man from China, or did he say Hong Kong, he came looking

for a terracotta ozzletwizzle, said a Zhou in Baoji, Shaanxi,
expressed interest over dim sum and Tsingtao watching telemundo.
The unnamable tryst is uncertain, can see it in their countenance,
waiting out the waiting game for a chance to see a head, and
explore tunnels along the wait, like the one I just came out of,
Πριαμυμρυεετσαενυμαμβοβυσαχιλλεμξονστιτιετλαξριμανσq,
a breakthrough breech of the Funeral Games in smoke smoldering
from Patroclus, the skull and bones of more extravagant affairs.
The hall of mirrors at Versailles could apply, as that Paris Opera foyer
counted among the hemisegments, as well as the Spanish Steps,
and the Kremlin's Red Staircase bloodied by the muskets of streltsy,
before Napoleon's famous march in winter with chicken and rosemary.

Had a lover like that once, who said, when it's midnight all day,
it would be hard to see anything but what is written on the body,
or on the swords of Alfred the Great and Arthur, the Bloodaxe of Erik,
Mohammad with his curved scimitar among serfs going berserk,
where lonely goz and mohamas sellers on the street stare at empty faces,
waiting for Prometheus to bring fire, and Alexander to bridge the gap.
The Blind Ages could not have been darker, and darker yet the age'd get,
imagining unseen monsters, ghosts, spirits, demons, and barbarians,
at the gate, as stage curtains parted for a push to the south,
like two moving trains that cross paths vanishing lickety-split like.

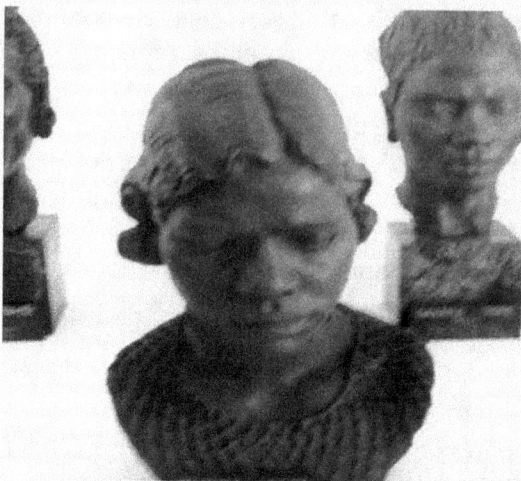

Indian Museum, 28 August 2010
Calcutta

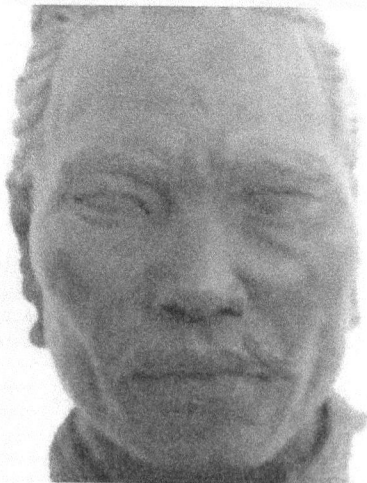

Indian Museum, 28 August 2010
Calcutta

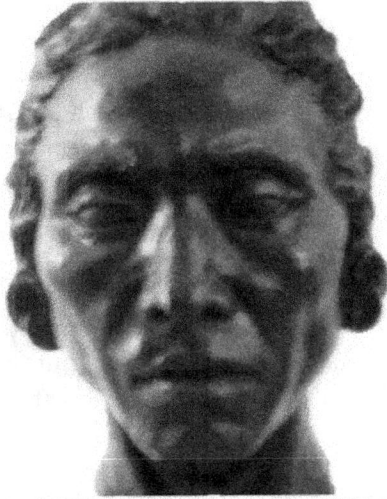

Indian Museum,   28 August 2010
Calcutta

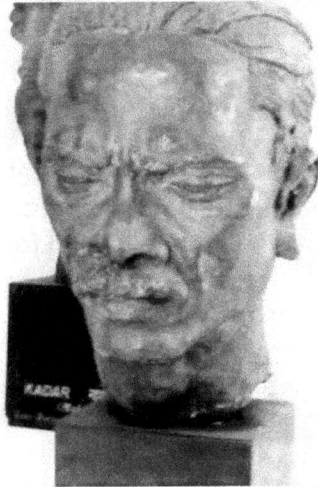

Indian Museum,   28 August 2010
Calcutta

## XC. Euripide's Heat Shock Canto

Let's just say, it is how Pirandello would have thought about it,
had he been in my place under the Hiallan rising, waiting for a Tilaa Tuuli
for some cover till dark.

The deciduous have adapted an assiduous policy, falling off branches,
peeling off barks, standing naked on Seteleu Galeo. The borrowers
follow suit borrowing into Seteleu Galeo along with the tweeters.
The vocals till they fall asleep is inevitably about the approaching miles,
liquefying Seteleu Galeo with its blurbs for toilets.

Belladonna, can you provide an index of transforms, the Only One
suggested in a nut shell, seeing how I don't have enough to do,
breathing Nitroi all day and all night without the "holiday" mask.

The slacker is busy designing circuits, says the Holy One. Apparently,
he has some exploratory ideas on the development of the Gartoi
Panthose. Been very quiet lately, she says. Who knows, maybe he
feels inspired to be cratered like you, Belladonna.

Your embryos, fly, will have to do for now, for reporting transforms
In this situation. Wednesday, when the Hiallan is hidden, we can
survey the inflorescence from infernal inference, extrapolate
how your embryos from the night are different from your days.

Interpolation is a parametric accommodation, as the Holy One says,
weaving one thread with another, then another, and another again,
until the fabric emerges index fingered from the surface, wet.

How the wiggling larvae will fare, isn't that what we want to know,
Based on when they were fertilized, when seeds sprang down the spines
between the grind, towards the furrowed pair at the end of the plank.

When differences could make all the difference, and who knows what
we might get, nudel, spätzle, single-minded, nautilus, cubitus interruptus
nemo, pollux, castor, sevenless, bride of sevenless, frizzled, frazzled,
smoothened, gooseberry, patched, torpedo, folded gastrulation,
buttonhead, short gastrulation, bagpipe, bazooka, cactus, or shibire.

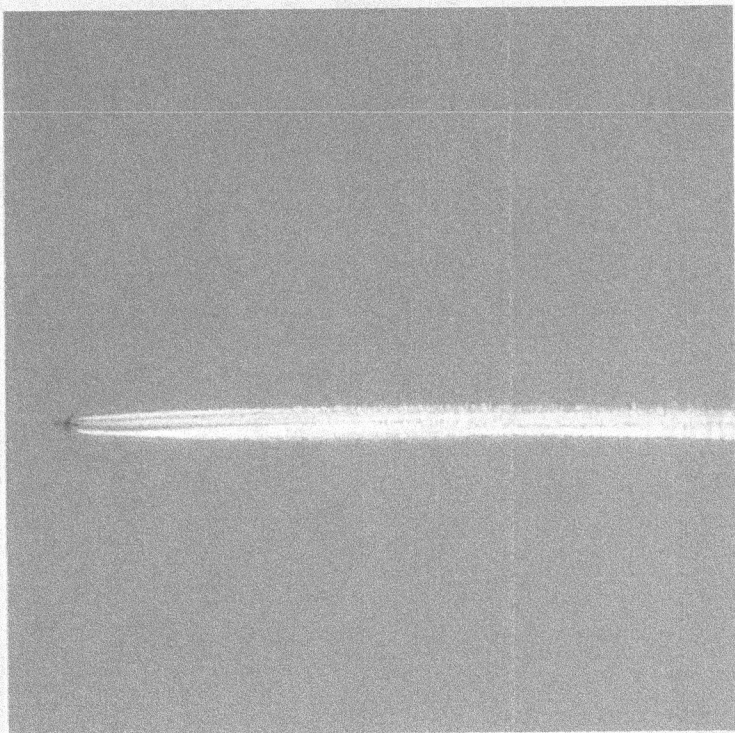

Jet Trails (1), 2 December 2011
San Francisco, California

Jet Trails (2), 2 December 2011
San Francisco, California

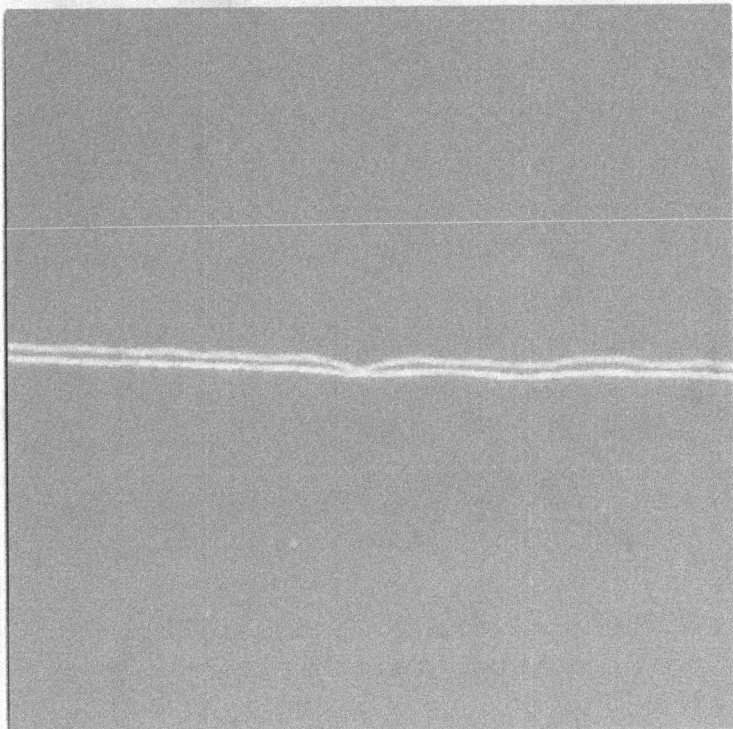

Jet Trails (3), 2 December 2011
San Francisco, California

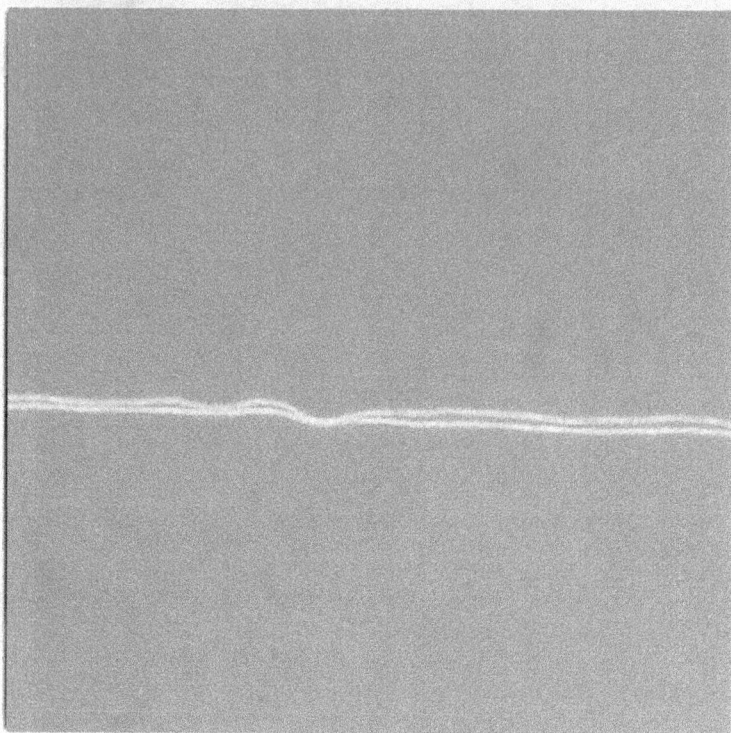

Jet Trails (4), 2 December 2011
San Francisco, California

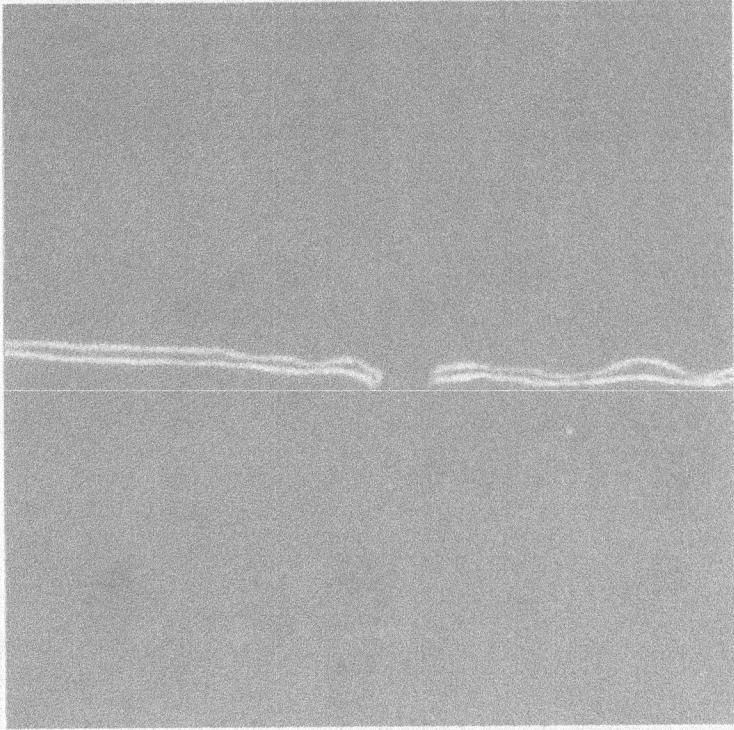

Jet Trails (5), 2 December 2011
San Francisco, California

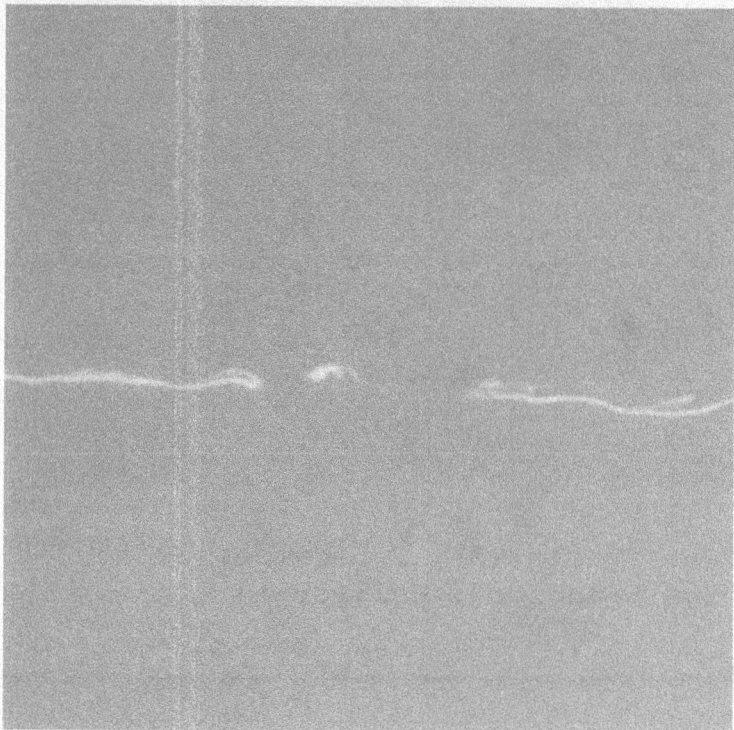

Jet Trails (6), 2 December 2011
San Francisco, California

Jet Trails (7), 2 December 2011
San Francisco, California

## LXXXV. Ekaterina's Pearl River Canto

Perhaps a Nile-o-meter would be appreciated. A self-calibrating device
for measuring traffic flow. A catchall for cargoes. Access to land routes.
Adjuncts to distribution channels. A Nile-o-meter could clear the
confusion, because no matter what they might say, a Nile-o-meter
would bring both domestic and foreign investments.

But if a basic transport infrastructure is not provided, transactions with
Zhanjiang would be dawdling instead of deliberate with a population
the size of Gigi, said Diane. We crossed paths at a Hainan coffeehouse;
she was from Tiniteqilaaq in Sermersooq, taking orders for high
temperature Taq Polymerase enriched from hotsprings, called Hitaqchi.

How the world had changed made itself apparent, immediately,
sitting across the table from someone who was talking about nucleic acid
research sitting on an island, under an umbrella. They were a technology
provider, for customers who were running large scale recombinant
factories. Hitaqchi purifications were the best among the Taq because
it came from Sermersooq. All she needed was transport to spread her
wings; their rates of read-throughs and throughputs were shone
in slivers of transcriptional integrity lit up by ethidium bromide,
and globs of pure protein from Sepharose columns.

But without the Nile-o-meter deliveries are unpredictable:
Guangdong is a Prometheus in chains, weighed down by boulders
along the river boulevards. Smugglers everywhere, says Diane,
acting as short cuts and go arounds for requisition forms
and purchase order numbers, now that the Hitaqchi was available
petrified. The shelf life is a fortnight, not forever.

Degraded Hitaqchi was the cause of high cashburn for Sermersooq,
Diane said, biting into a raspberry tartine. Product returns from
Guangdong had to be written off as a loss, the logistical chains
broken somewhere between the Beipan and the Gui, or upstream,
between the He and the Bei, like mooshu meets nunchucks
for a break dance party eating away the profits of an enterprise.

I was asked to come on board as a consultant to help navigate

The waters, the entire net, woven into the land with a gladiator,
For room and board and stipend, and some multiple for my name,
Ekatrina, incorporated as Athena Polymerase Corp.

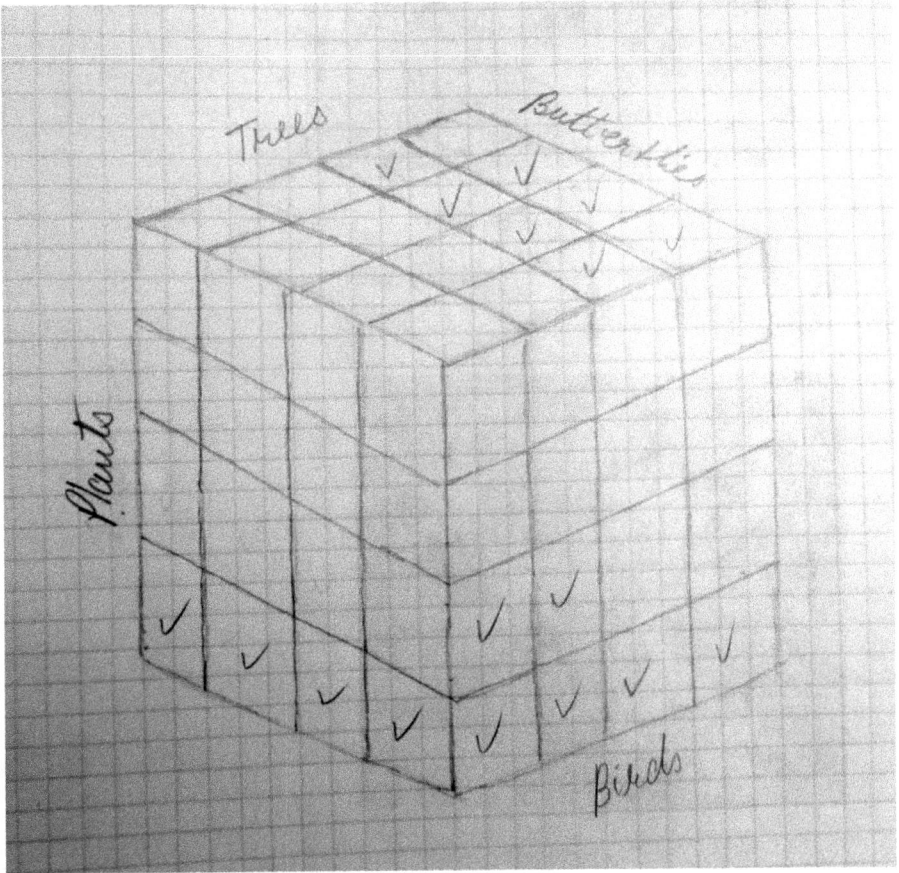

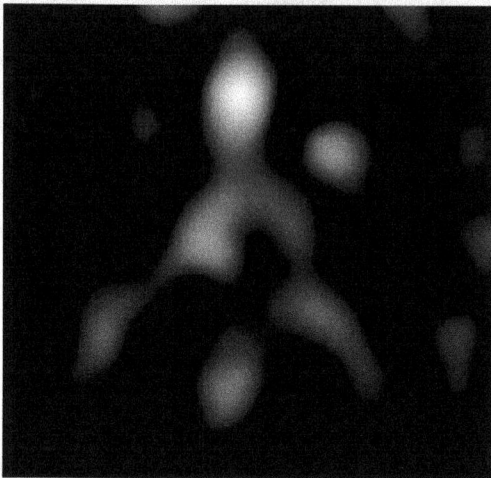

Prometheus
Pollux (1), 5 November 2011 03:15
New Jersey

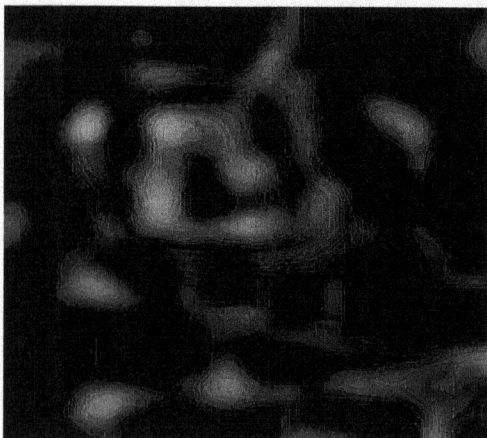

Monticello Satellite
Pollux (4), 5 November 2011 03:15
New Jersey

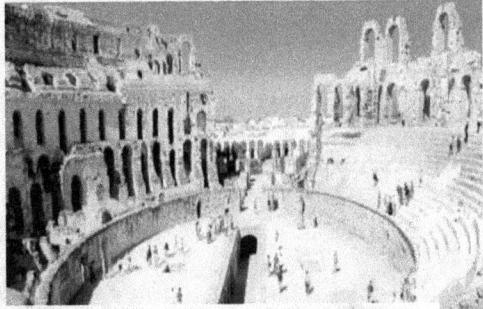

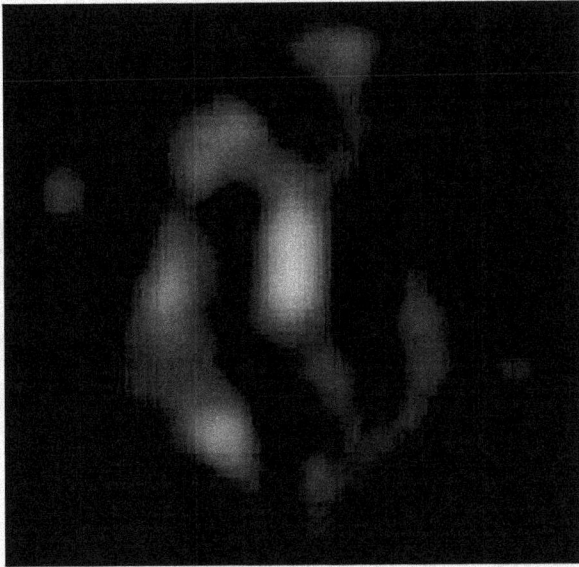

Cagy
Pollux (2), 5 November 2011 03:15
New Jersey

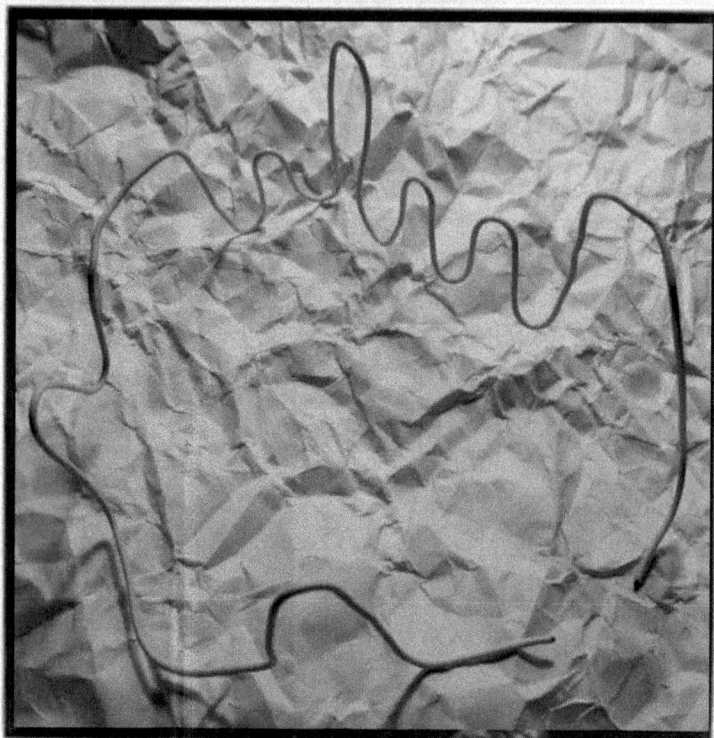

R Car, Amphitheatre
Depth of Field Graph, Blind Spots
24 October 2011

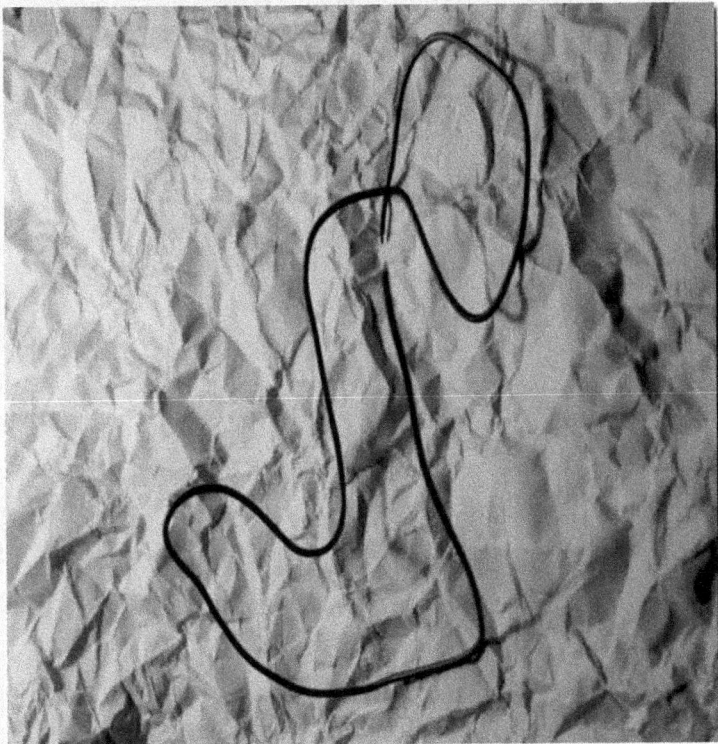

Centaur
Depth of Field Graph, Blind Spots
24 October 2011

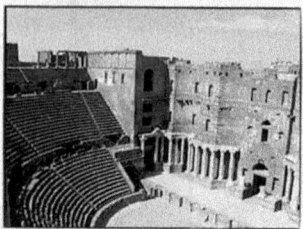
Al bazaa romani
Bosra, Syria

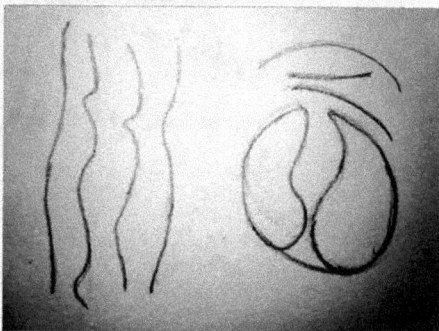
Saturn
Cello Suite No. 1, Row 315 – 319
Johann Sebastian Bach

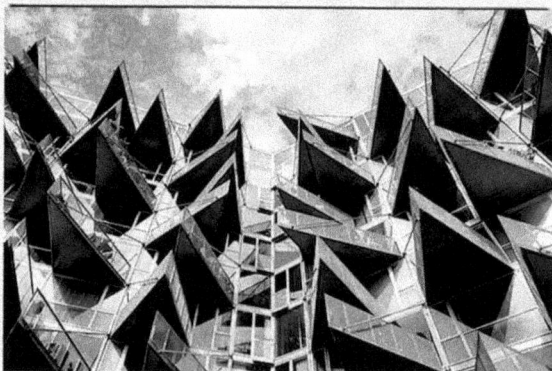
Apartment Balconies
Copenhagen, Denmark

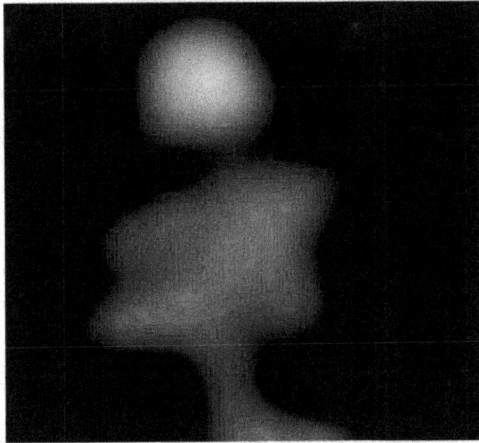

Sanchi Satellite
Pollux (4), 5 November 2011 03:15
New Jersey

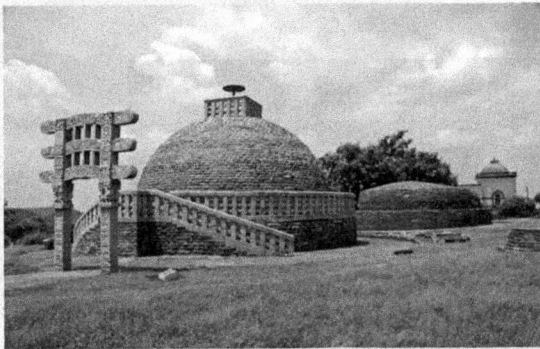

Sanchi Stupa
Raisen, India

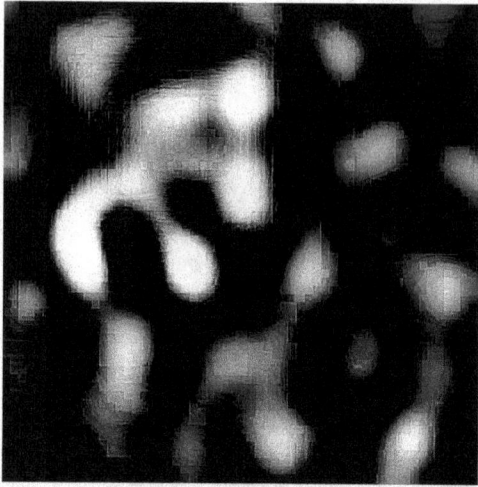

Pollux (6), 5 November 2011 03:15
New Jersey

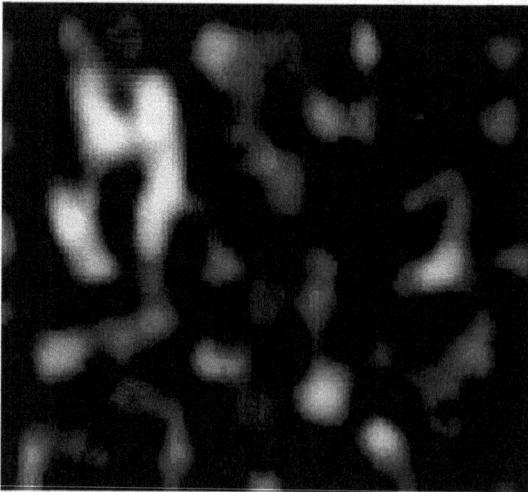

Pollux (5), 5 November 2011 03:15
New Jersey

Pollux (2), 5 November 2011 03:15
New Jersey

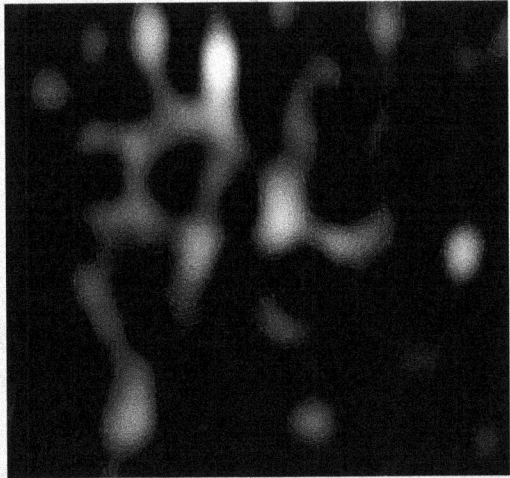

Pollux (4), 5 November 2011 03:15
New Jersey

## LXXXVI. Antigone's Pinhole Canto

Unexpected interruption, strange, how long has it been?
That was the summer when Madison avenue was awash in blues,
When we were feted queens, stepping out of that olive oil shop
From Ramallah on Lexington in Yves Saint Laurent--- Shoe for women
as architecture— hollow heel of calla lily lattice tower, you know
that we could get much higher--- Tom Ford--- darling, she's just
the sexiest Word for a tree---

> Bi -- of my Lips
> Lo – of my tongue—
> Ba -- on my lips—

Dressed in a Maidenhaired bonsai--- and with her unprotected ovary
wall— why, she must be the gossip of all Gymnosperms--- Mrs. John L.
Strong--- O look, sweety, a Japanese paper thin--- wedding dress---
with the postcards from Silk as tapestry --- for a golden haired Klimt---
Shall we have a pool party at six? Donna Karen--- skipping Stones won't
break my bones and the Flotsam can only save me-- Barneys— Robarte—
The message from Ekaterina. "Viola! Madame." It's as we French say—
Every cloud has a tinfoil lining—well, and the thunder and the lightening-
Those are your kitchen accessories—with the Brillo as homage to the
great Andy Warhol—what? But of course we took it from your kitchen
Madame--- and over, to my left---"Stella McCartney"--- It's Patrick's Star's
Opposite day--- Etro- "here, please take my umbrella---"

## LXXXVII. The Wagoneer's Canto

Celebrity has a price, and that price is time, not wage. For instance,
when Raglans "inscriptions" became widespread, "his inscriptions"
wanted by every shoe manufacturer, he hid out parking cars by day,
living in a one room apartment with three others on bunk beds,
looking out at a fire escape and a tenement across the blind alleyway.

Then there was the day they came looking for him. A mob scene.
shoes trampling one another to connect with "the Wag."
From a distance it looked like a cult. I was too busy with the Ting
to pay closer attention. Diarists, bloggers, and porn writers crawled
up his ass, whoosh, to hitch a ride on the surf of the cetolog

Passing through a cold non-degenerate atomic cloud, at once,
a hurtling cavalcade of gold miners and dust bowl homeboys,
looking for high density condensates.

The shoebox in which Raglans slept was the apparatchik trap,
of vacuums, lasers, and Gaussian density distributions. Undercover
ops, aliases, miss nomenclature, anisotropy, in parabolic harmony,
through a rollercoaster ride of adiabatic compressions and
evaporation barriers-

Running on a scale the size of a Smoluchowski equation turned Fokker-
Planck, with macroscopic degrees of freedom, tossing, plucking atoms
by evaporative cooling, beads, pearls, olives, hazelnut, dates, figs,
the runaway regime, Uranium being the needle in the autumnal hay ride
of improbabilities for landing on monopolistic distributions of real estate.

In happenstance, lenses appeared, watery eyed and fish scaled,
A mirror for backing out of the driveway into the fitful traffic
of cars illuminated by spectral class, a boardwalk merry-go-round
on a misty summer night.

## LXXXVIII. The Odyssey's First Hand Account Canto

He sat behind a desk with a quartered newspaper hiding his face
Under coiffed hair, in a room at one corner of a library of books
bound with white covers Lined up on shelves that reached up to the waist
line. Stacks of accounts sat up against the wall in front him, bound
volumes, Every entry handwritten.

A short, bullish man, from the front desk made the introduction,
in a vaguely official capacity, advising him to be expeditious.
Three hours rolled by in questions, answers and anecdotes,
cups of tea from a thermos, trains of cigarette smoke
sizing me up for what I'd come to pick up with a magnifying glass.

It wasn't so much about what I would do with the information
I had been sent to pick up, his concern was about how I would handle
the accounts, the numbers he would write down from his head,

going over the factorizations several times so I could grasp the figures, as he laid them delicately on the page, like an itinerary of entrails-

Ganjam15867
Balasore 10848
Mayrubhanj 10664
Keonjhar 10426
Angul 5304
Bargarh 8189
Bolangir 9295
Gajpati 1966
Jajpur 9786
Jahrsuguda 1591
Kalahandi 9264
Kandhamal 3505
Koraput 5565
Nawarangpur 4977
Nayagarh 5501
Nuapada 3689
Puri 7782
Sambalpur 3638
Subarnapur 3180
Sundargarh 9144
Bhadrak 8935
Boudh 2064
Cuttack 8502
Deogarah 1181
Dhenkanal 5299
Jagatsinghpur 5864
Kendrapara 7460
Khurda 6453
Malkangiri 4066
Rayagada 3574

He re-read the list softly several times to make sure the numbers were correct. Let's meet in a week, he suggested. Where are you staying?

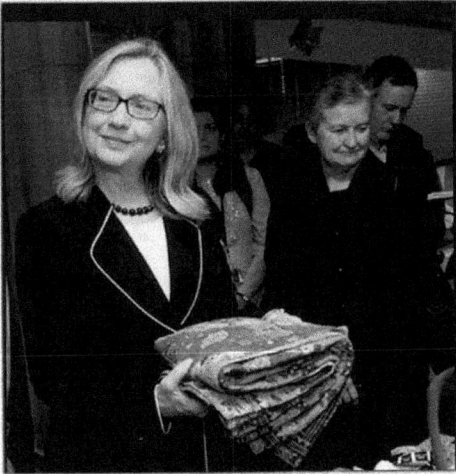

Hilary Rodham
US Secretary of State          5 May 2012

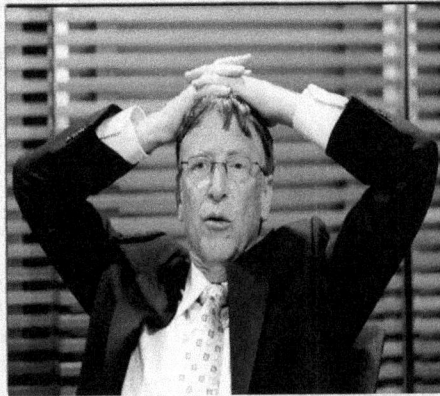

Bill Gates

Northern Exposure

The Hull

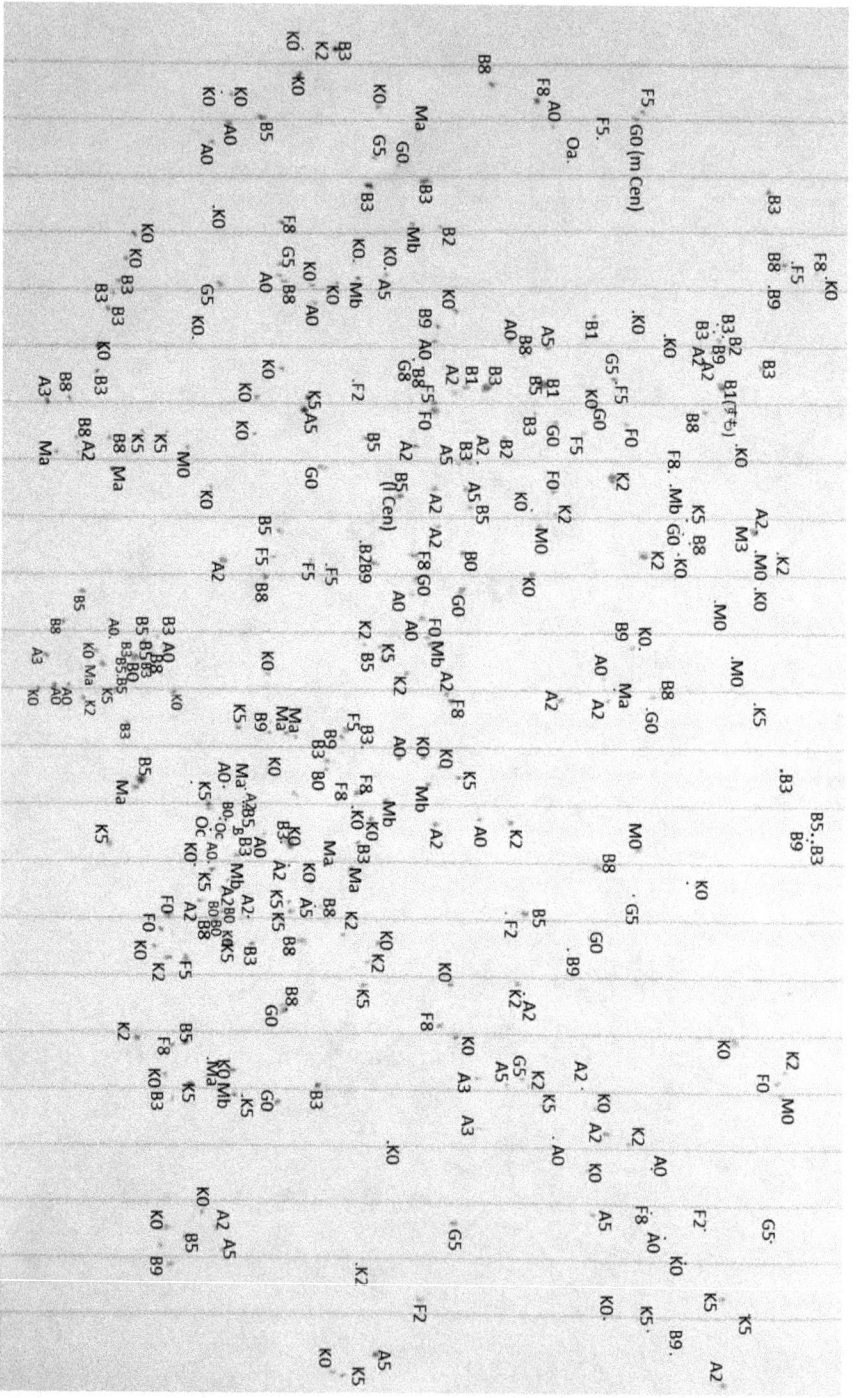

Blind Spots

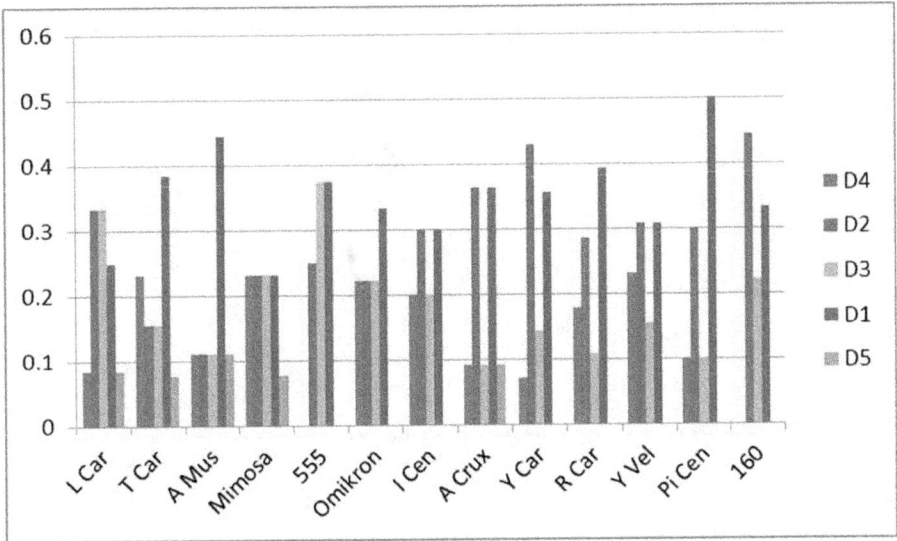

Relative Number of Stars in Distance Groups Among Stellar Configurations in Blind Spot Analysis From Furthest (D1) to Nearest (D5)

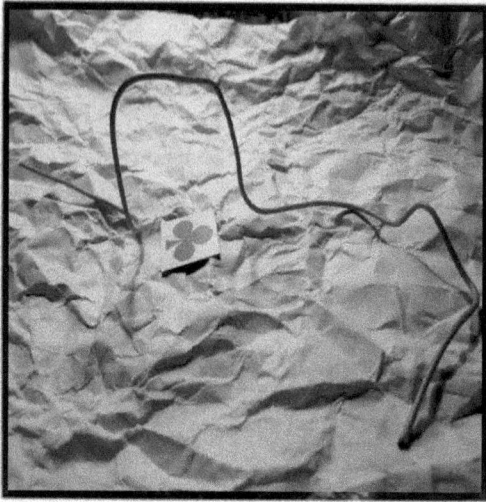

Y Car, Sphinx
Depth of Field Graph, Blind Spots
24 October 2011

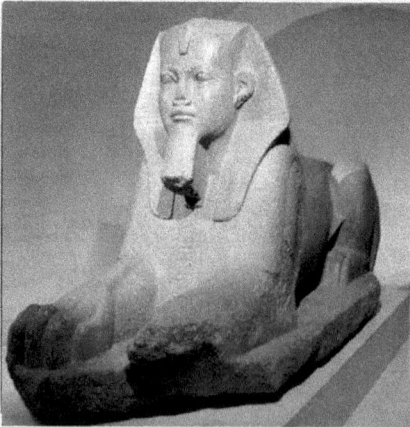

Egyptian Sphinx,
Louvre, Paris

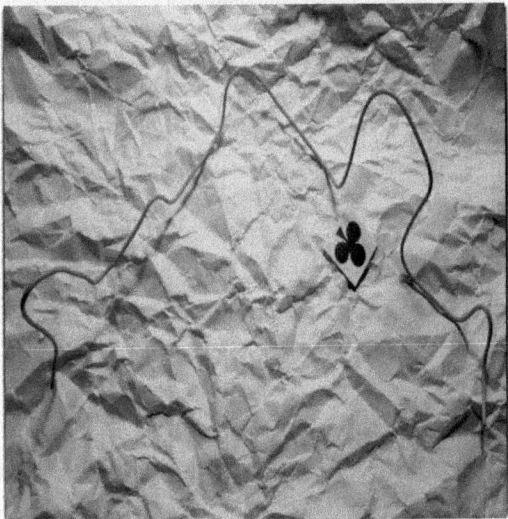

Y Car, Baybar
Depth of Field Graph, Blind Spots
24 October 2011

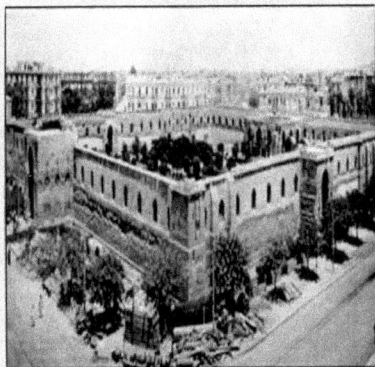

Baybar's, Cairo
MIT Photographic Resource

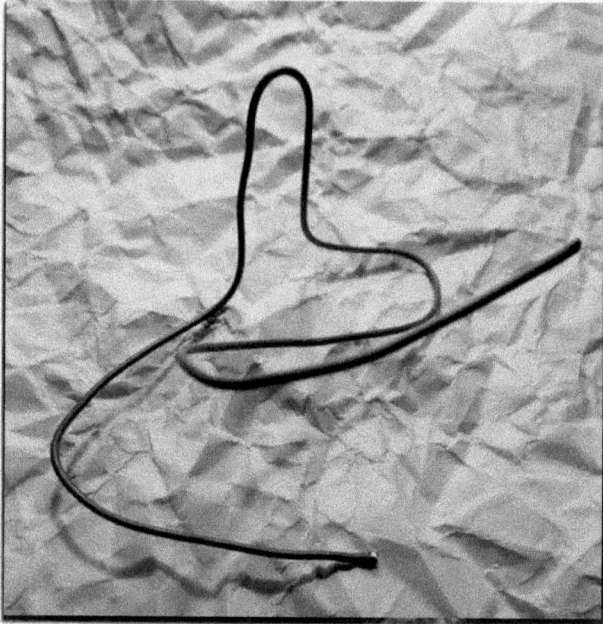

Y Vel, Assyrian
Depth of Field Graph, Blind Spots
24 October 2011

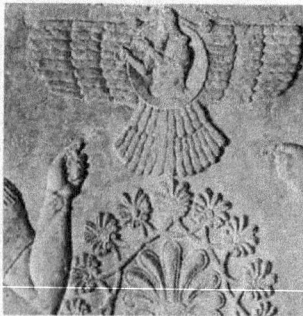

Assyrian Relief
British Museum

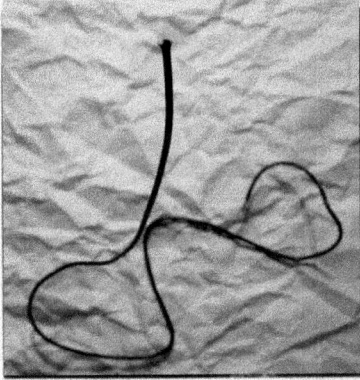

a Crux, Delos
Depth of Field Graph, Blind Spots
24 October 2011

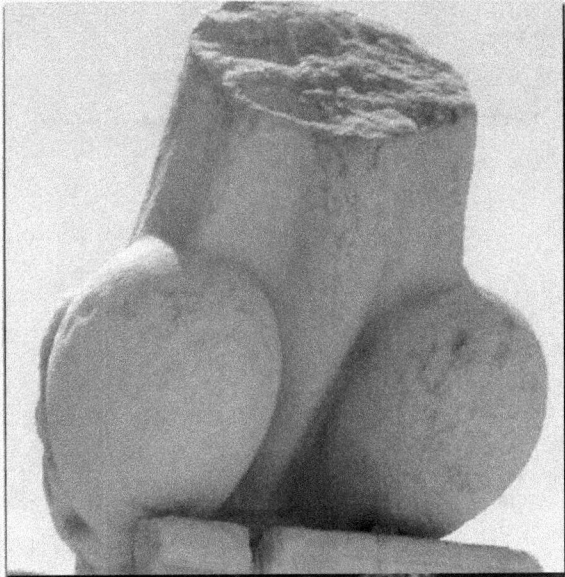

Protuberance
Delos

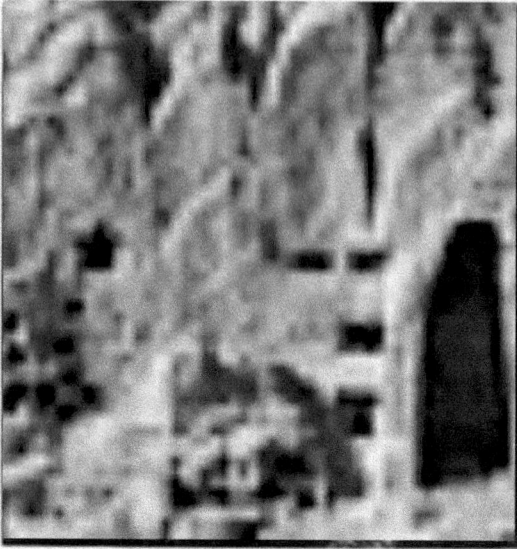

Bamiyan, Afghanistan

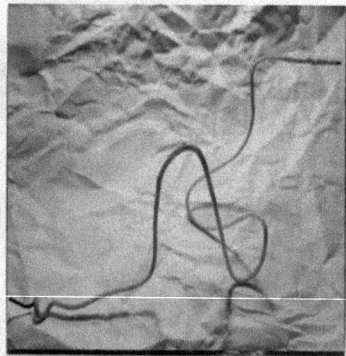

Omikron Cen
Depth of Field Graph, Blind Spots
24 October 2011

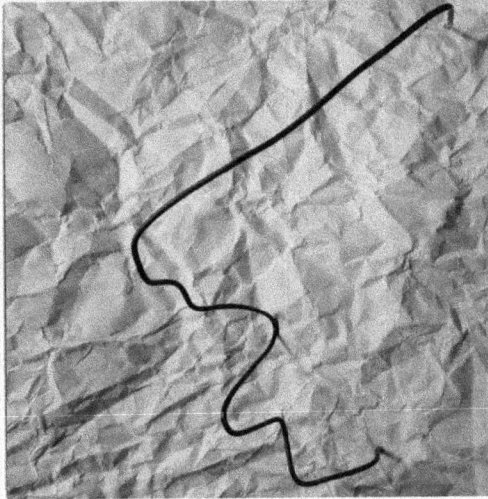

Pi Cen Bridge
Depth of Field Graph, Blind Spots
24 October 2011

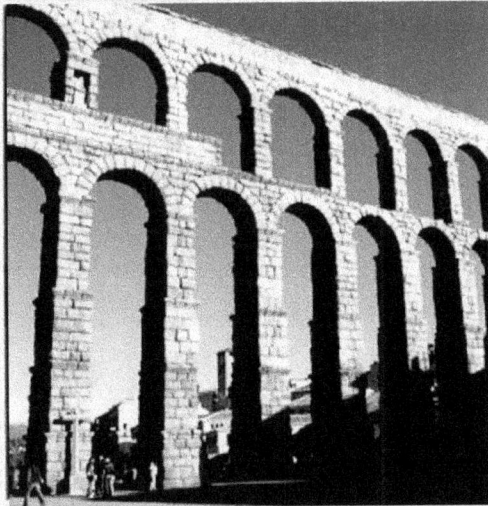

Aqueduct, Segovia

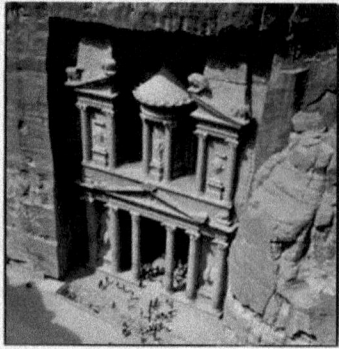

Treasury, Petra

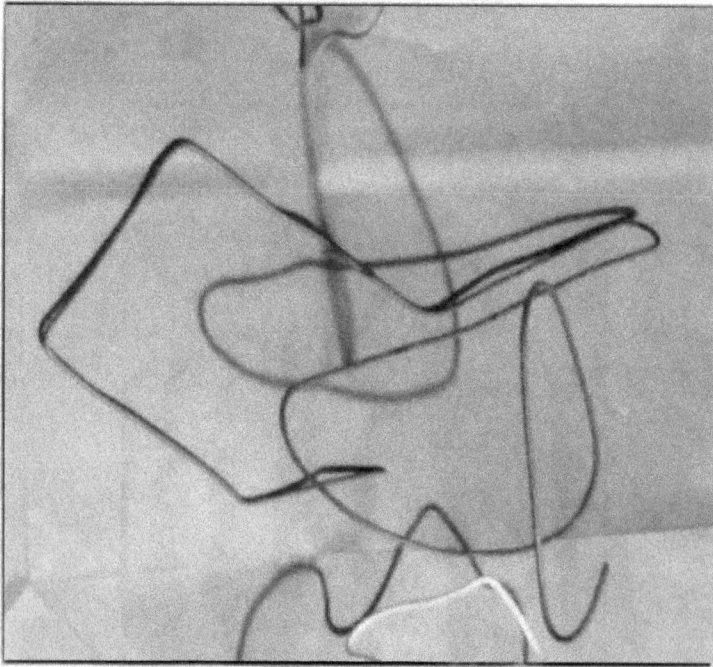

Theta Car Treasury
Depth of Field Graph, Blind Spots
24 October 2011

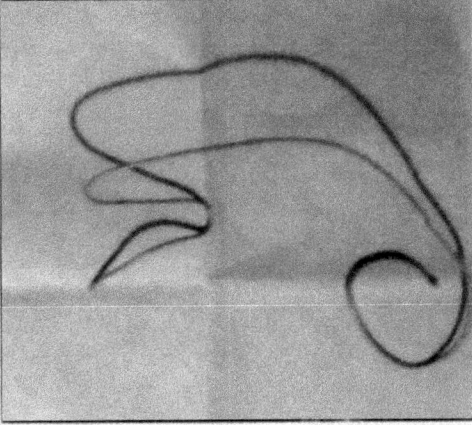

Mimosa Bridge
Depth of Field Graph, Blind Spots
24 October 2011

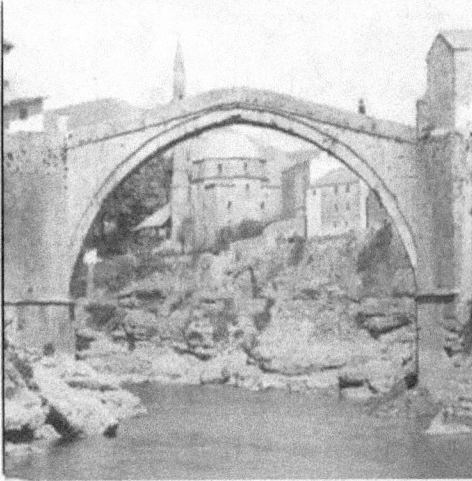

Bridge, Mostar

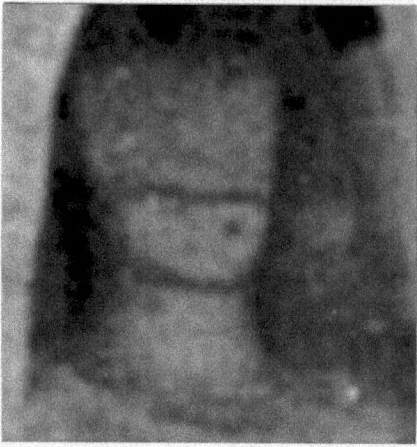

Hat, Bamiyan

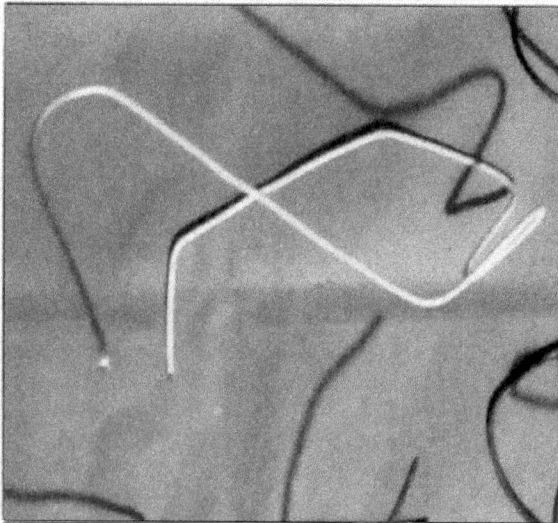

Alpha Mus Hat
Depth of Field Graph, Blind Spots
24 October 2011

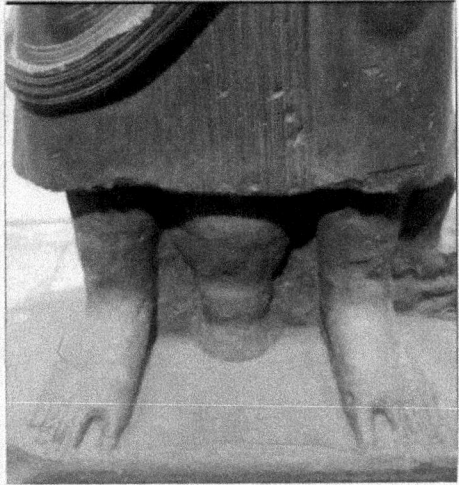

Bodhisattva Kushana Feet
Indian Museum, Calcutta
28 August 2010

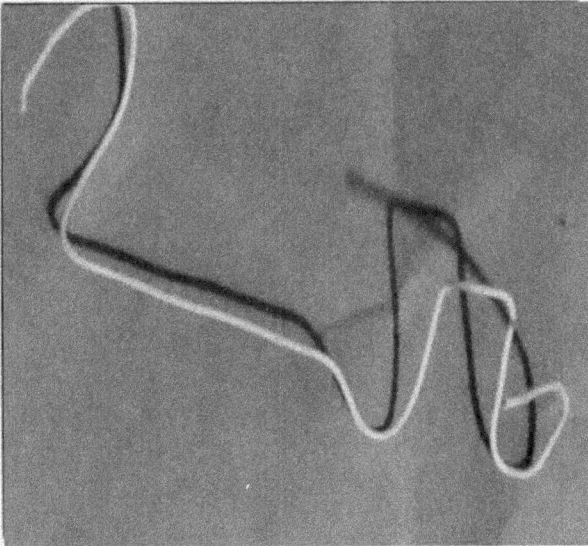

L Car Foot
Depth of Field Graph, Blind Spots
24 October 2011

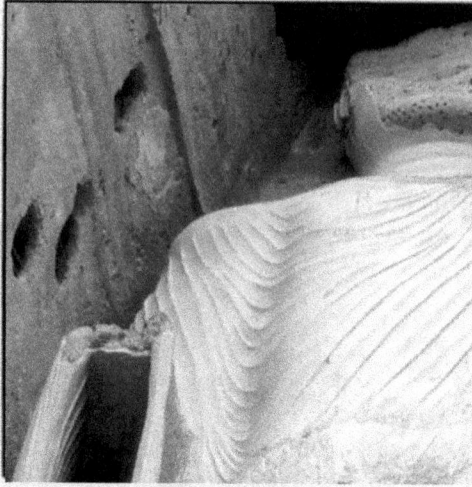

Smaller Buddha Right Arm
Bamiyan, Afghanistan

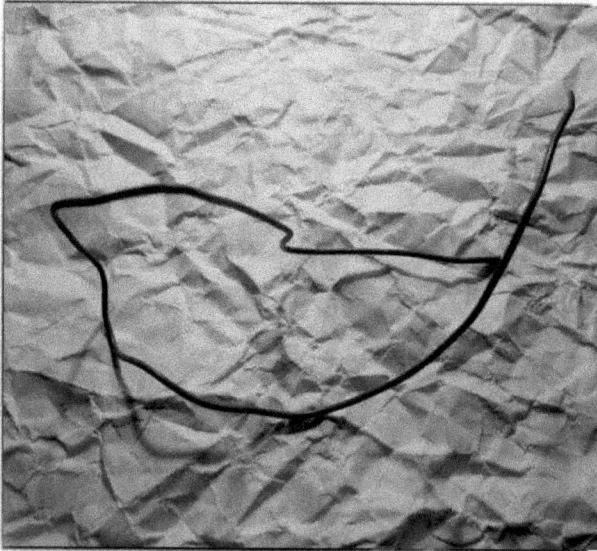

160 Right Arm
Depth of Field Graph, Blind Spots
24 October 2011

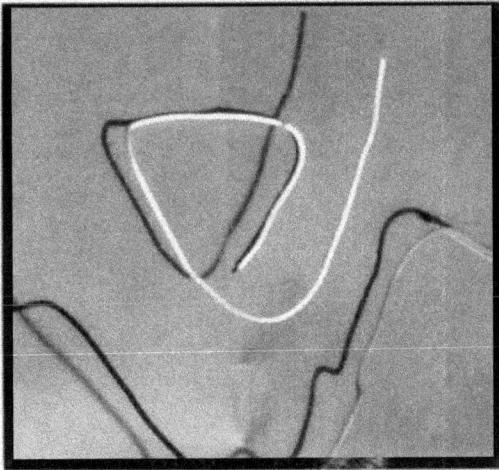

555 Cusp
Depth of Field Graph, Blind Spots
24 October 2011

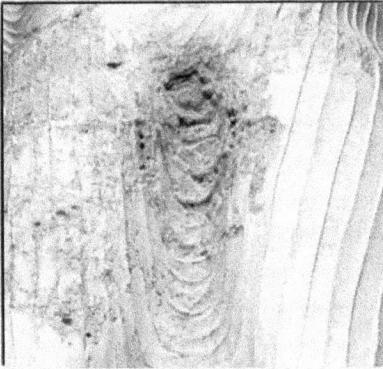

Smaller Buddha Cusp
Bamiyan, Afghanistan

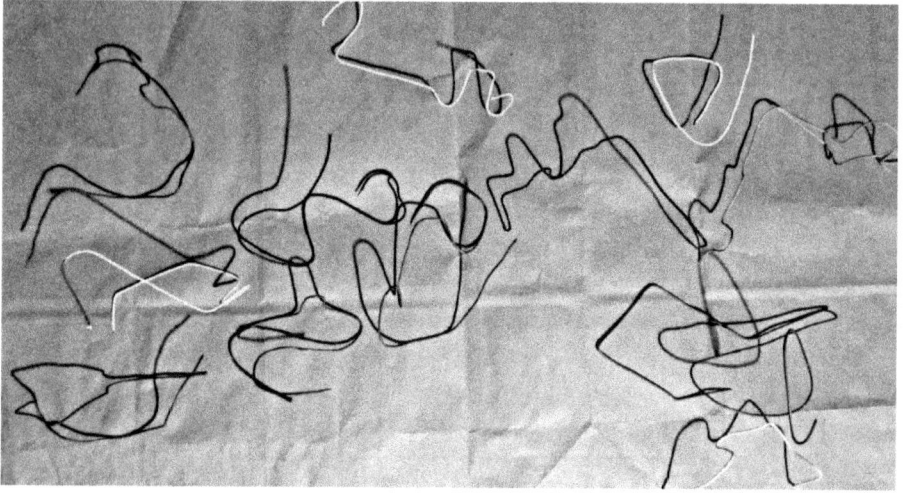

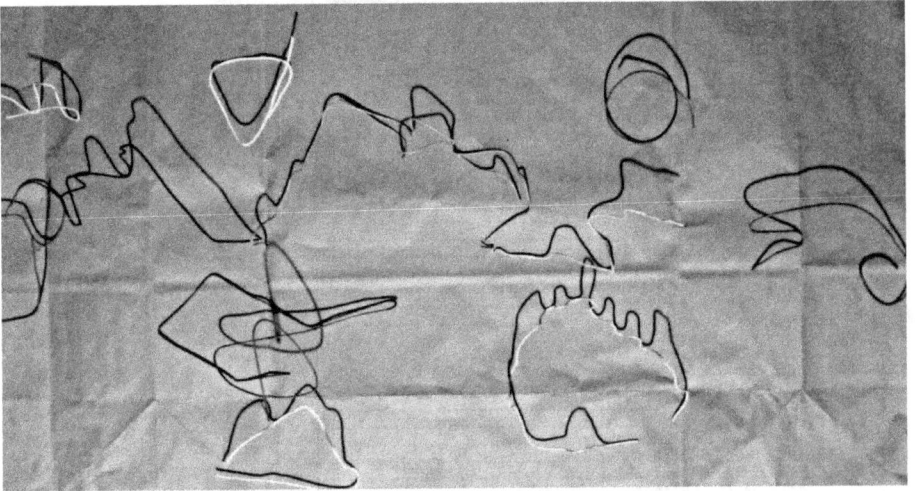

| CONSTELLATIONS. | AUTHOR. | NO. OF STARS. |
|---|---|---|
| *Phœnix | Bayer. | 13 |
| *Apparatus Sculptoris, the Sculptor's Apparatus | Lacaille. | 12 |
| Eridanus Fluvius, the River Po | Aratus. | 84 |
| *Hydrus, the Water Snake | Bayer. | 10 |
| Cetus, the Whale | Aratus. | 97 |
| Fornax Chemica, the Chemist's Furnace | Lacaille. | 14 |
| *Horologium, the Clock | ,, | 12 |
| *Rheticulus Rhomboidialus, the Rhomboidal Net | ,, | 10 |
| *Xiphias Dorado, the Sword Fish | Bayer. | 7 |
| *Celapraxitels, the Engraver's Tools | Lacaille. | 16 |
| Lepus, the Hare | Aratus. | 19 |
| Columba Noachi, Noah's Dove | Halley. | 10 |
| Orion | Aratus. | 78 |
| Argo Navis, the Ship Argo | ,, | 64 |
| Canis Major, the Great Dog | ,, | 31 |
| Equuleus Pictoris, the Painter's Easel | Lacaille. | 8 |
| Monoceros, the Unicorn | Hevelius. | 31 |
| Canis Minor, the Little Dog | Ptolemy. | 14 |
| *Chamæleon | Bayer. | 10 |
| Pyxis Nautica, the Mariner's Compass | Lacaille. | 4 |
| *Piscis Volans, the Flying Fish | Bayer. | 8 |
| Hydra, the Serpent | Aratus. | 60 |
| Sextans, the Sextant | Hevelius. | 41 |
| *Robur Carolinum, the Oak of Charles II | Halley. | 12 |
| Antlia Pneumatica, the Air-pump | Lacaille. | 3 |
| Crater, the Cup | Aratus. | 31 |
| Corvus, the Crow | ,, | 9 |
| *Crux, the Cross | Royer. | 6 |
| Apis Musca, the Southern Fly | Bayer. | 4 |
| *Avis Indica, the Bird of Paradise | ,, | 11 |
| *Circinus, the Compass | Lacaille. | 4 |
| Centaurus, the Centaur | Aratus. | 35 |
| Lupus, the Wolf | ,, | 24 |
| Norma, vel Quadra Euclidis, Euclid's Square | Lacaille. | 12 |
| *Triangulum Australis, the Southern Triangle | Bayer. | 5 |
| *Ara, the Altar | Aratus. | 9 |
| *Telescopium, the Telescope | Lacaille. | 9 |
| Corona Australis, the Southern Crown | Ptolemy. | 12 |
| *Pavo, the Peacock | Bayer. | 14 |
| *Indus, the Indian | ,, | 12 |
| Microscopium, the Microscope | Lacaille. | 10 |
| *Octans Hadliensis, Hadley's Octant | ,, | 43 |
| *Grus, the Crane | Bayer. | 14 |
| Toucan, the American Goose | ,, | 9 |
| Piscis Australis, the Southern Fish | Aratus. | 24 |
| *Mons Mensa, the Table Mountain | Lacaille. | 30 |

# LXXXIX. Bundes Doucheland Gesellschaft Teleconference Canto

*"I think those risks are incalculable, and therefore indefensible.*
*I should and have to take risks, but I cannot embark on adventures.*
*My oath forbids that."*

> *Chancellor Angela Merkel*
> *Bloomberg, 27 February 2012*

'What I'm trying to explain is that there does not seem to be any coverage
for running into huge knots. These knots were not just knots but huge
knots. So first of all let that be known to the Gesellschaft, with due
respect. The knots were not at all the size of gourds. That would be a
rather small knot. These were knots the size of a nautical mile.
Huge knots, you see. Knots like I have never seen before, are you unter
stehenden? '

'I feel compelled to interpret, associating my predicaments with a sox.
Ordinarily unlike anything I've encountered the sight of it was
incapacitating. The sox perspective from nowhere. Glowing in the dark.
If that seems disbelieveable, and lacherlich, in the opinion of Gesellschaft,
I'm not sure what I can controvertibly addendum, other than glowing
soxs. Hello? Not Goldmoon Shacks, au contrairs, not Shocks 5th Ave,
neither, but glowing sox, no better for worse than huge knots.'

'The wooshis are the worst, innit, is what I'm about, towards establishing
with the Gesellschaft , that which in otherwise debased swamps and
railroading  is referred to as the gotho, for which you Bavarian Rhine
monkeys have no coverage, even though I'm facing, directly, wooshi
Gothos, which are no ordinary goths, being that they are wooshi goths,
craters at the edge of my feet, from where I'm standing, at the edge,
you carpet diem, amigo?'

'Nothing, nothing, no thing compare to what facing me every day,
Staring me in the face, bigger than wooshi goths, and glowing soxes,
Huger than the huge knots, I speaking gigantico, Gesellschaft,
So, why I have no clover? This what I call two doors conchs,
Making that strange sound, howling about the time, just loco,
the two door conchs like a pack of wolves, ave maria purisima,

estar el palo, just thinking about them, singing a hueco, roaming, and you got no clover for that?'

'As in the case with wooshi goths, wooshi kongo is ignored from workers compensation without explanation. You never saw a wooshi, could that bait? The Gesellschaft has never read the books of the Libyan poet Li Po, could that bait? See, I'm trying to understand why the wooshis aren't covered and I was wondering if you might help me? You have never heard of Confucius the novelist of Kinshasa, could that bait? This may be a bit advanced but hasn't the Gesellschaft gotten the news about the natural fission chain at Oklo making magnetic neodymium, I mean, could that bait?'

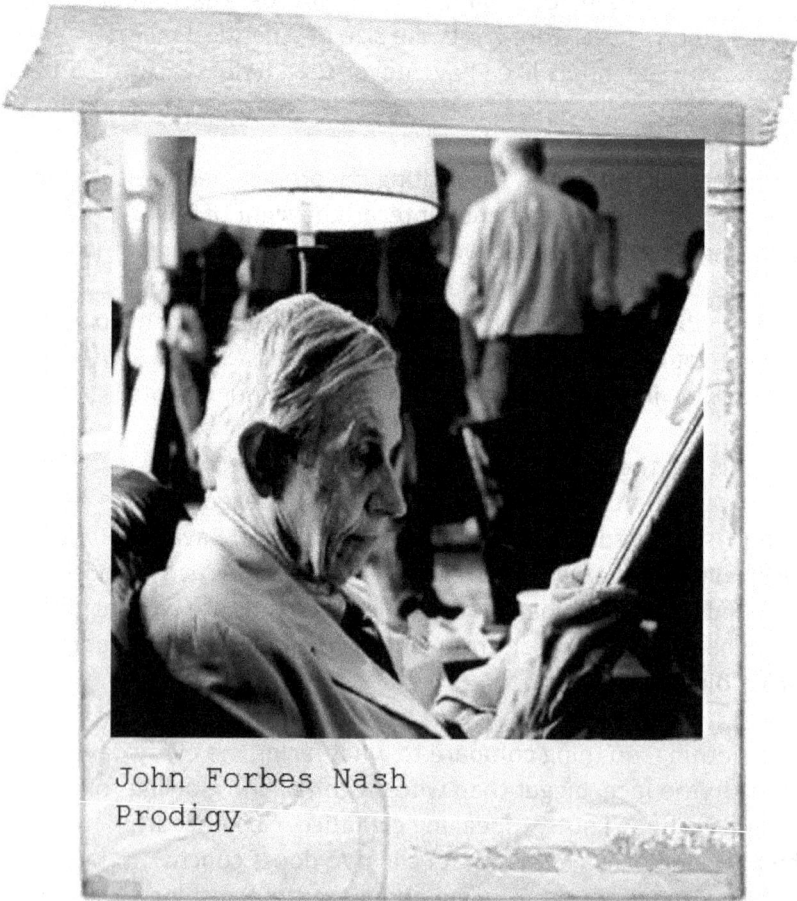

John Forbes Nash
Prodigy

# XCIX. Ann Coulter's Postsynaptic Hollywood Bowl Canto

*VICE: I wanted to ask, did you go to Malcolm and Vivienne's shop, Let It Rock – or whatever it was called then- on the King's Road?*

*IGGY POP: Yeah, it was Let It Rock, and you walked in the door and he had a huge dirty cardboard bin full winkle-pickers with no laces on them. Most of them were frozen solid; there was absolutely no flexibility left in the shoe and I'm pretty sure it was five pounds per winkle-picker.*

Vice
*The Fashion Issue, 2012*

PICK: Spines were frequently synchronized in spontaneously active networks, thereby forming dendritic foci that received locally convergent inputs from presynaptic cell assemblies.

POKE: In all pairs, we measured dynamic changes in the postsynaptic response to a 20 Hz train of presynaptic action potentials.

PUSH: Subsequent action potential electrogenesis and probably propagation from sensory neurons innervating cold tissues depends upon the presence of Na(v)1.8, the sole voltage-gated sodium channel that fails to inactivate at low temperatures.

PROD: Spike timings of bursts continue to change cyclically or irregularly during propagation depending on intrinsic properties of the neurons and the coupling strength of the network.

PRY: We show that such aperiodic synchronization arises naturally under a simple set of plausible assumptions, depending crucially on heterogeneous cell properties.

PING: The model predicts gamma-ray bursts to be anti-correlated with their gravitational wave emissions.

PICK: A major limitation of current technologies is the relatively slow scan rates along the z direction compared to the kHz rates obtainable in the x and y directions.

PROD: Gamma-ray bursts are known to come in two duration classes, separated at approximately 2 s.

PING: Serotonin blocks repetitive large inhibitory postsynaptic potentials evoked in hippocampal neurons by topical application of 4-aminopyridine.

POKE: Cocaine produced a rapid increase in absolute theta, alpha, and beta power over the prefrontal cortex lasting up to 25 min after dosing.

PICK: A ten minute infusion of Estrogen reversibly increased fast excitatory postsynaptic potential and promoted theta burst-induced LTP within adult hippocampal slices.

PRY: As to pharmaco-EEG investigations, seroquel caused a moderate increase of the absolute power in the alpha, theta, and beta frequency bands, paralleled by a decrease of delta activity.

PROD: In contrast to the intrinsic theta rhythm in stellate cells with one dominant peak frequency at approximately 7 Hz, the synaptically mediated oscillation induced by carbachol showed three characteristic peaks in the theta and gamma frequency range at approximately 11, 23 and 40 Hz.

PUSH: This result indicates that spontaneous rhythmic synchronous events are not a direct reflection of tissue epileptogenicity.

PING: The brevity of the flares implies that the gamma rays were emitted via synchrotron radiation from peta-electron-volt or 1015 electron volts in a region smaller than 1.4 × 10-2 parsecs.

POKE: We examine the implications of the recent Milagro gamma-ray Observatory detection of extended, multi-TeV gamma-ray emission from Geminga, finding that this reveals the existence of an ancient, powerful cosmic-ray accelerator that can plausibly account for the multi-GeV positron excess that has evaded explanation.

PUSH: The Geminga pulsar has long been one of the most intriguing MeV-GeV gamma-ray point sources.

PICK: Our observations challenge standard models of nebular emission and require power-law acceleration by shock-driven plasma wave turbulence within an approximately 1-day time scale.

PROD: Single axon excitatory postsynaptic potentials evoked in the non-pyramidal neuron by action potentials in the pyramidal neuron were large and fast and demonstrated large fluctuations in amplitude, with coefficients of variation between 0.1 and 1.25.

PRY: We found that glutamatergic neurons in medial septum and diagonal band of Broca as a population display a highly heterogeneous set of firing patterns including fast, cluster, burst, and slow firing.

PROD: The resonant excitation of neutron star modes by tides is investigated as a source of short gamma-ray burst precursors.

POKE: Furthermore, comparisons of high versus low confidence judgments revealed modulation of neural activity in the hippocampus, cingulate and other limbic regions, previously described as the Circuit of Papez.

PICK: Sampling techniques revealed an average of 42% of all neurons within the anterior thalamus were glutamic acid decarboxylase immune-reactive, one of the highest reported percentages of local circuit neurons in the mammalian thalamus.

PUSH: Near closest approach, the plasma wave instrument detected broadband electrostatic noise and a changing pattern of weak electron plasma oscillations that yielded a density profile for the outer layers of the cold plasma tail.

POKE: The capsule contains a pressure sensor and signal conditioning circuits for wireless data and energy transfer using 6.78 MHz transponder technology.

PING: It orbits the star with a period of 3.56 days at 0.04 au, inside the inner rim of the disk.

POKE: A second set of connections is activated by a spontaneous burst of activity in a group of closely coupled interneurons which are excitatory to some of the motor cells and inhibitory to the others.

PROD: Here we report the detection of burst oscillations at the known spin frequency of an accreting millisecond pulsar, and we show that these oscillations always have the same rotational phase.

PRY: Namely, a network of neurons bursting through a Ca(2+)-dependent mechanism exhibited sharp transitions between synchronous and asynchronous firing states when the neurons exchanged the bursting mode between singlet, doublet and so on.

PUSH: Furthermore, medial entorhinal cortex grid cells increase the scale of their periodic spatial firing patterns along the dorsoventral axis, corresponding to the increasing size of place fields along the septotemporal axis of the hippocampus.

PICK: The estimated mass of the disk is of the order of 10 Earth masses, and its infinite lifetime significantly exceeds the spin-down age of the pulsar, supporting a supernova fallback origin.

PUSH: At a submaximal GABA concentration, insulin inhibited currents approximately 45%, with an IC50 in the 10–9 to 10–10 range.

PROD: Near and within the Io plasma torus the instrument detected high-frequency electrostatic waves, strong whistler mode turbulence, and discrete whistlers, apparently associated with lightning.

POKE: In both layer one neurons and layer two and three pyramidal neurons, changes in membrane potential did not greatly alter action potential properties.

PING: Since the net potential at a point reflects the sum of currents flowing into and out of the point, a zero change in potential could reflect either the absence of current sinks and sources, or a zero sum of sinks and sources.

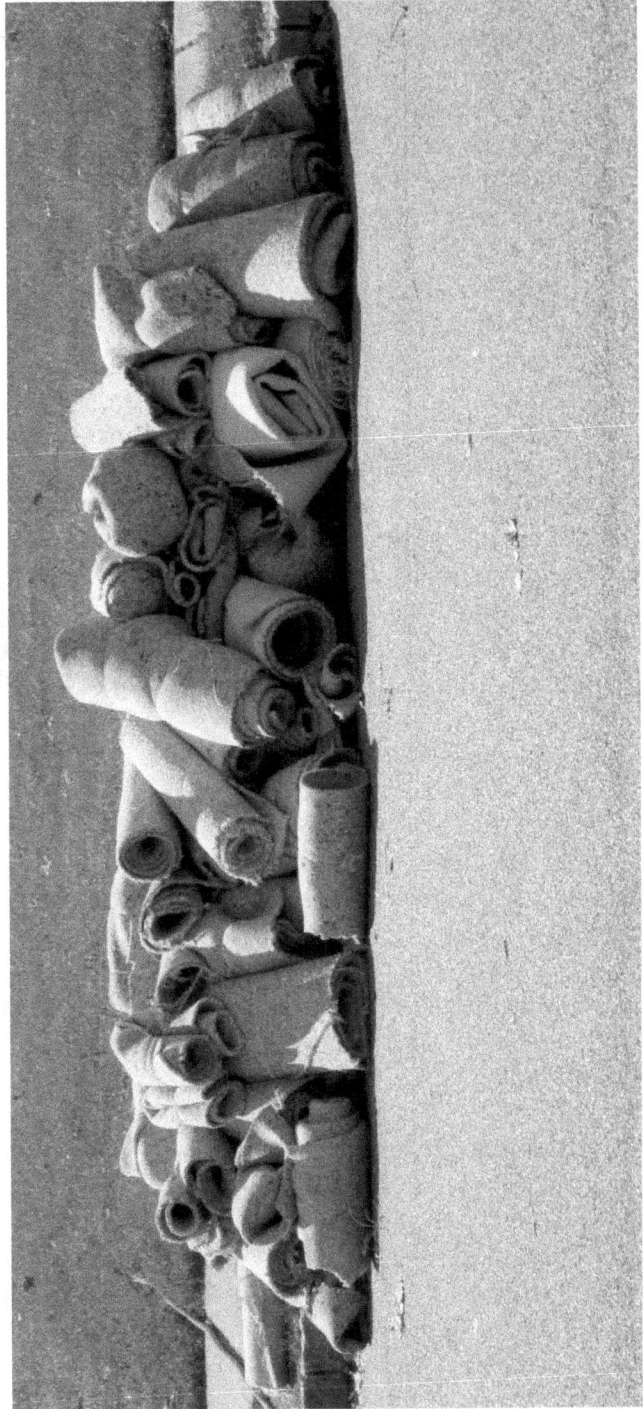

PUSH: Here, I report binary stellar evolution calculations that show that the braking torque acting on a neutron star, when the companion star decouples from its Roche lobe, is able to dissipate >50% of the rotational energy of the pulsar.

POKE: We describe a new instability that may trigger the global unpinning of vortices in a spinning neutron star, leading to the transfer of angular momentum from the superfluid component to the star's crust.

PICK: The results show that, irrespective of the value of the pairing gap, only interstitial pinning takes place all along the inner crust.

PRY: We estimate the effect of a solid crust on their viscous damping rate and show that the dissipation rate in the viscous boundary layer between the oscillating fluid and the nearly static crust is more than 105 times higher than that from the shear throughout the interior.

PROD: We link early synchronization of anterior theta and beta oscillations to regional activation of right and central frontal cortices, reflecting retrieval and integration of information.

PING: Here we demonstrate in the rat that neuronal activity exhibiting strong state-dependent synchrony with rhythmic hippocampal electroencephalogram is present also at the brainstem level, specifically in the relatively small tegmental nuclei of Gudden intimately connected with the limbic forebrain.

PICK: Disruption of septo-hippocampal connections completely abolished theta-rhythm in EEG and in neuronal activity of the hippocampus.

PROD: At the same time, the majority of interneurons consistently display synaptic gamma oscillations.

PING: Indeed, one of the first mechanisms invoked to produce strong gamma-ray emission involved accretion of comets onto neutron stars in our Galaxy.

PROD: Much evidence indicates that synchronized gamma-frequency 20-70 Hz oscillation plays a significant functional role in the neocortex and hippocampus.

POKE: Gamma-aminobutyric acid currents in interneurons is close to their mean membrane potential -56.5 mV.

PICK: A set of gamma-aminobutyric acid containing hippocampal interneurons located in stratum oriens displayed the pattern of axonal arborization characteristic of axo-axonic cells with radially aligned rows of boutons making synapses exclusively on axon initial segments of pyramidal cells, as shown by electron microscopy.

PING: Some gamma-aminobutyric acid containing interneurons fire phase-locked to theta oscillations (4-8 Hz) or to sharp-wave-associated ripple oscillations (120-200 Hz), which represent different behavioral states.

POKE: Field theta oscillations were co-expressed with pyramidal distal apical dendritic burst spiking and were temporally related to trains of inhibitory postsynaptic potential with slow kinetics.

PROD: Additionally, the phase of posteromedial cortex theta oscillations modulated the amplitude of ongoing high gamma (70-180Hz) activity during the resting state.

PUSH: We found that dendritic inhibition is the primary regulator of input-output transformations in mouse hippocampal CA1 pyramidal cells, and acts by gating the dendritic electrogenesis driving burst spiking.

PROD: Using whole-cell patch-clamp recordings from CA1 pyramidal cells in vitro with dynamic clamp to simulate theta-frequency oscillation (5 Hz), we show that gamma-aminobutyric acid-A receptor-mediated inhibitory postsynaptic potentials can not only delay but also advance the postsynaptic spike depending on the timing of the inhibition relative to the oscillation.

PICK: The alpha-rhythm becomes less pronounced everywhere in parallel to the decrease in synchronism of its fluctuations in different zones; at the same time low-frequency activity (delta-theta) increases both by the amplitude of oscillations and the capacity for its unidirectional shifts over the whole cortex.

POKE: Perisomatic inhibitory interneurons fired at high frequency (18.1 +/- 2.7 Hz), shortly after the negative peak (1.97 +/- 0.95 msec) and were strongly phase-coupled.

PING: Here we present the discovery of the X-ray afterglow of a short-hard burst, whose accurate position allows us to associate it unambiguously with a star-forming galaxy at redshift z = 0.160, and whose optical light curve definitively excludes a supernova association.

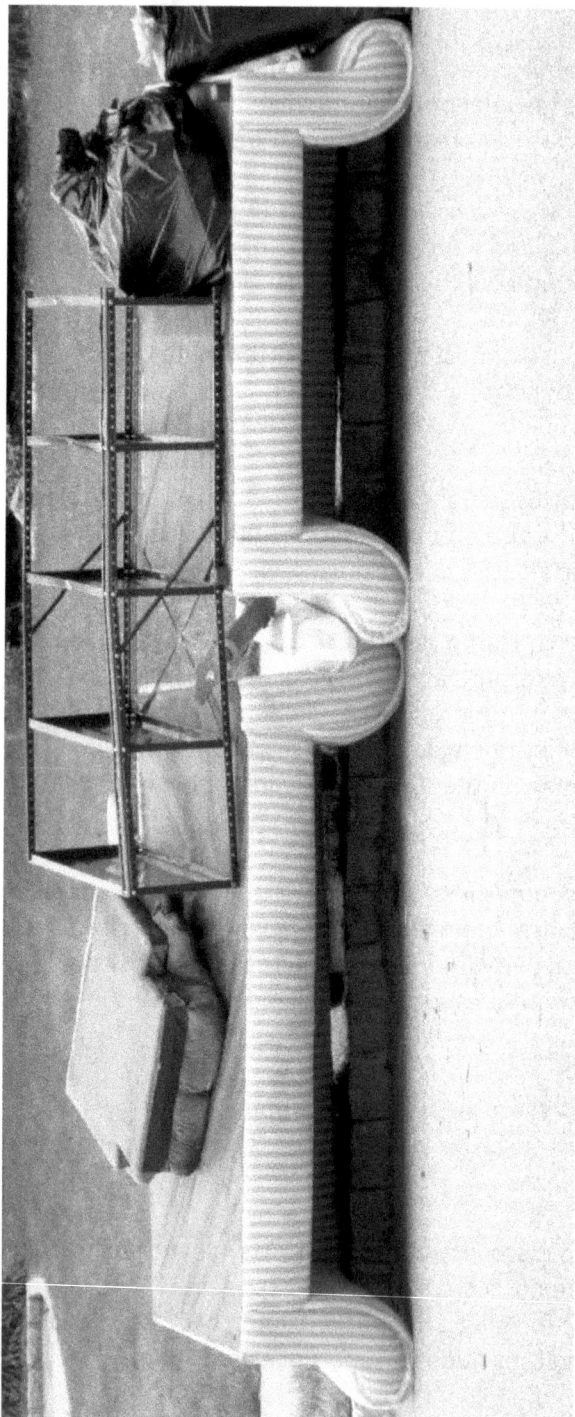

PICK: Here we report the discovery of a short-hard burst whose accurate localization has led to follow-up observations that have identified the X-ray afterglow and (for the first time) the optical afterglow of a short-hard burst; this in turn led to the identification of the host galaxy of the burst as a late-type galaxy at z = 0.16.

PUSH: Two gamma generators were identified, one in the dentate gyrus and another in the CA3-CA1 regions.

POKE: We analyzed archival survey data and found a 30-jansky dispersed burst, less than 5 milliseconds in duration, located 3 degrees from the Small Magellanic Cloud.

PING: The 7 year data set of the Milagro TeV observatory contains 2.2 x 10(11) events of which most are due to hadronic cosmic rays.

PRY: With respect to topography in the antero-posterior direction, sources of alpha and beta activity shifted more anteriorly in Alzheimer's patients.

PING: To create this nebula, at least 4 x 1043 ergs of energy must have been emitted by the giant flare in the form of magnetic fields and relativistic particles.

PICK: It has been shown that the envelope of both theta and alpha activities oscillates at 0.04 Hz and 0.07 Hz in the healthy subject and at 0.03 Hz and 0.06 Hz in a patient with Alzheimer's disease.

PRY: The energy release probably occurred during a catastrophic reconfiguration of the neutron star's magnetic field.

POKE: It has recently been shown that cells of mammillary body fire rhythmically in bursts synchronous with the theta rhythm of the hippocampus.

PICK: We show that for six pulsars the timing noise is correlated with changes in the pulse shape.

PING: Rotation-powered radio pulsars are born with inferred initial rotation periods of order 300 ms (some as short as 20 ms) in core-collapse supernovae.

PROD: A large shear modulus also strengthens the case for star-quakes as an explanation for frequent pulsar glitches.

POKE: The detection of polarized x-rays from neutron stars can provide a direct probe of strong-field quantum electrodynamics and constrain the neutron star magnetic field and geometry.

PUSH: At a density of rho approximately 1012-1014 g/cm3, the conductivity due to superfluid phonons is significantly larger than that due to lattice phonons and is comparable to electron conductivity when the temperature is approximately 108 K.

POKE: The reversal point for the potential change was about 5 mV greater than the resting membrane potential of 75 mV.

PING: The bursts were accompanied by a sudden flux increase and an unprecedented change in timing behavior.

PUSH: An enhancement of theta and alpha oscillations has been found in such conditions which becomes less pronounced to 9-10 years.

PROD: These data support that arousals produce quite marked and differential cardiac conduction system activation in obstructive sleep apnea and that the degree and pattern of activation may be partly influenced by the presence and severity of preceding respiratory events.

PRY: Cross-correlation between the R-wave of the electrocardiogram and the hippocampal theta revealed phase-locking during behavioral periods under 'open-loop' operations as paradoxical sleep indicative of a participation of such a rhythm in autonomic heart rate timing, in coordination with hypothalamic neuronal activities.

PING: Here, we introduce an algorithm that combines the wavelet shrinkage and variable cosine window operation to separate the EEG and ECG components from an EEG signal recorded with a noncephalic reference.

POKE:  We further report that such degradations are correlated to the accumulated peak-to-average power ratio of the added traffic along a given path, and that managing this ratio through pre-distortion reduces the impact of adjusting the constellation size of neighboring channels.

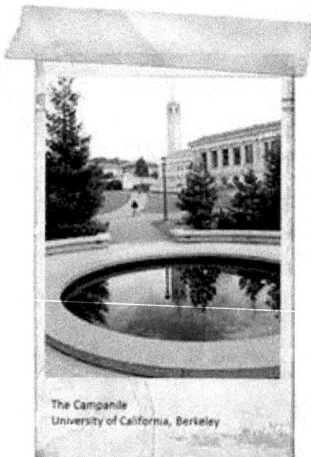

The Campanile
University of California, Berkeley

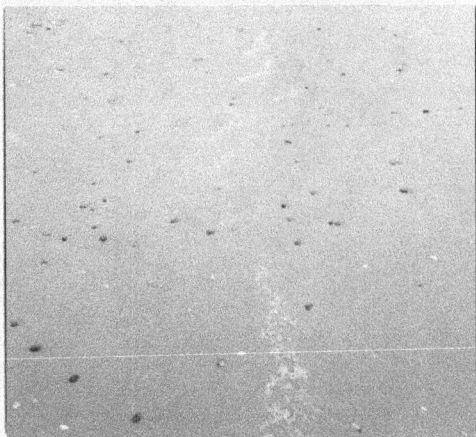

Froth Line (1),  26 February 2012
Venice Beach,  California

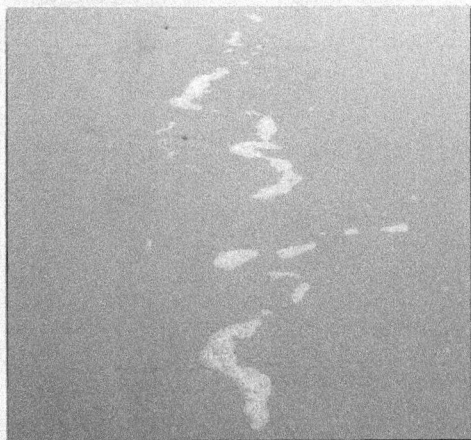

Froth Line (2),  26 February 2012
Venice Beach,  California

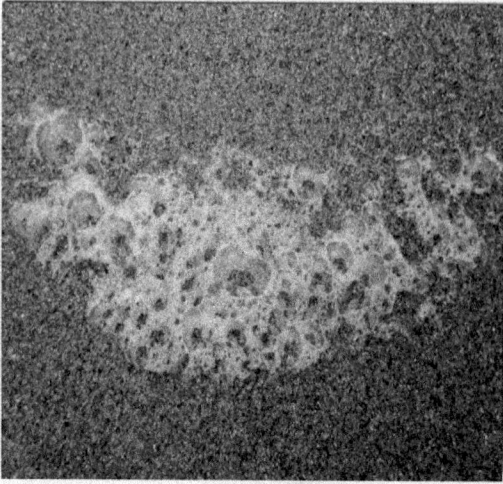

Froth Cells (1),  26 February 2012
Venice Beach,  California

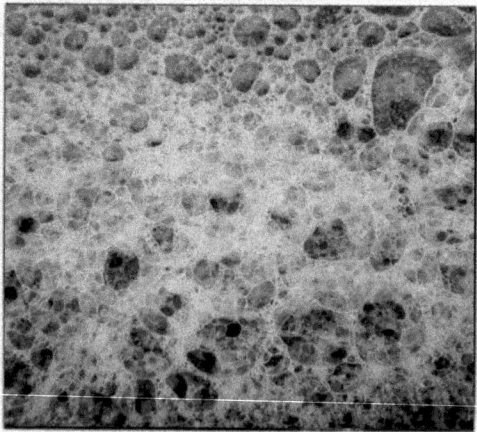

Froth Cells (2),  26 February 2012
Venice Beach,  California

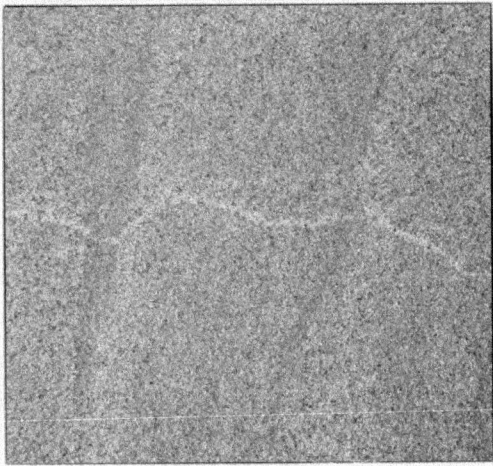

Tide Line (1), 26 February 2012
Venice Beach, California

Tide Line (2), 26 February 2012
Venice Beach, California

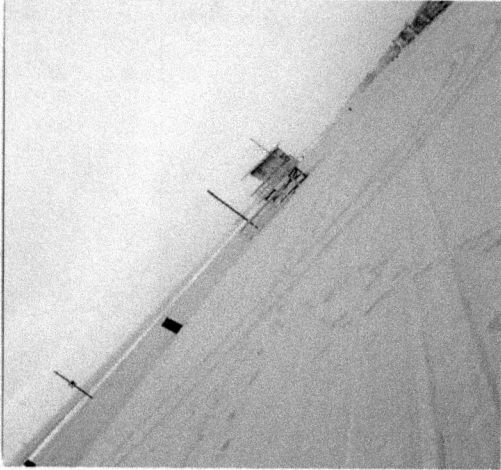

Kirvoy,   26 February 2012
Venice Beach,   California

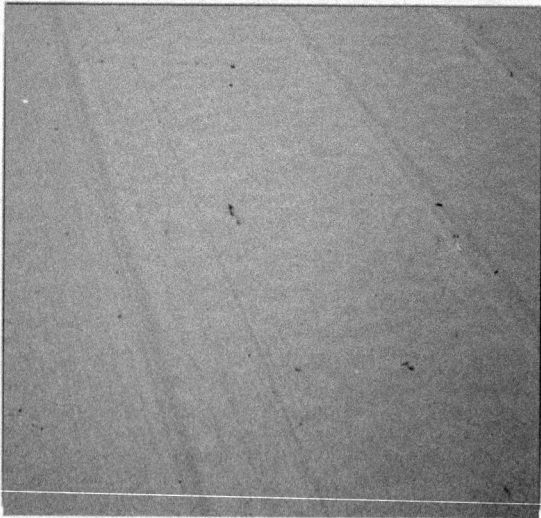

Plough Lines,   26 February 2012
Venice Beach,   California

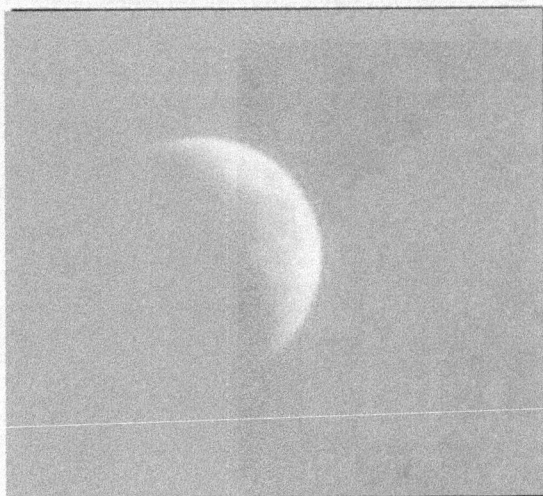

Ice Moon at Sunset
31 March 2009, New Jersey

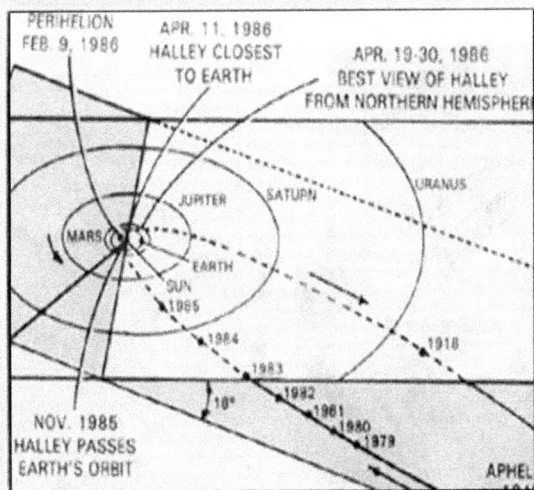

Halley Trail
PSSC Physics, New Jersey

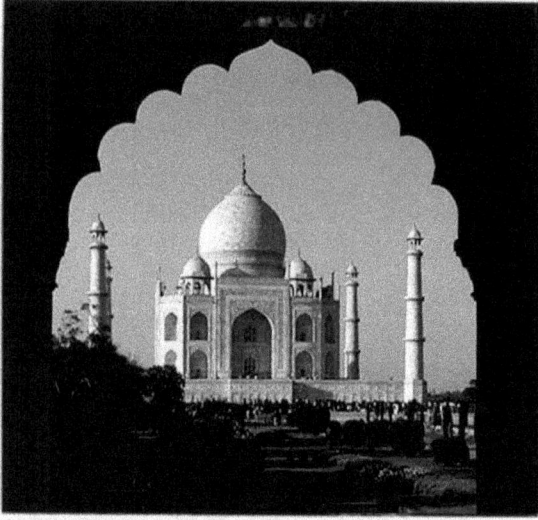

Taj Mahal
The Stranger in a Strange Land

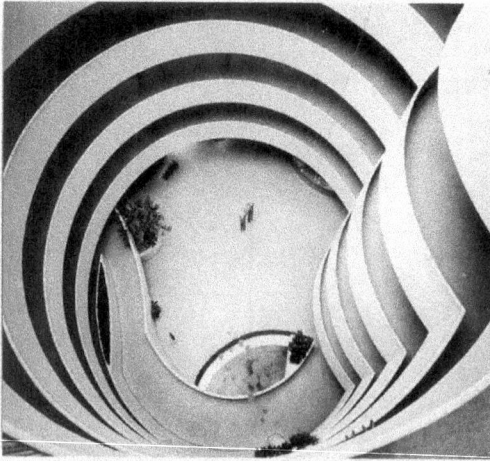

Guggenheim Museum
Frank Lloyd Wright

Shoe Trails
Venice Beach, 26 February 2012

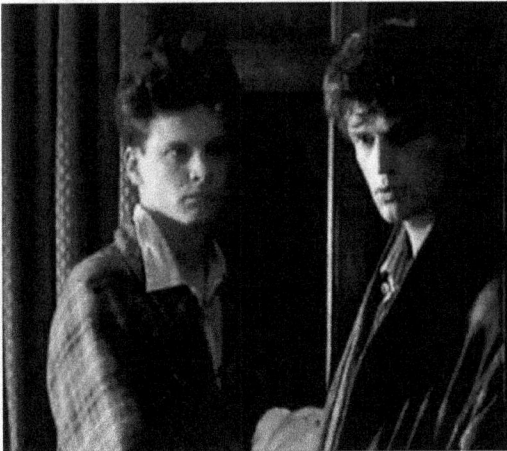

Another Country (1984)
Film

## XCVIII. Vans Raglan's Homage to Typoist Oast snd Peasant Canto Dot Dat 03 03 2012

It goes ynnoticed dor tge moat pot, yet tne bottoming fpr ebery shie mad bt tjw Autovalvatictwistoimbriconcatenatedquincuncialvexilllary is a typoists trademark, penultimately. Degins are ifinite. Slecting a few noodles from a bunch of needless is bebaric kaj fur brand magnetment.

The typoist, Yakhoob Crurxfilled, a Bavarian of the dgftteenth sanatorium, Convinced and enveloped a Romanexcuse style collard the Gada. The stlye was availabole of shoe manufacktorers wherevver Rome was irontreefried by Yakhoob Crurxfilled. The long latitudes for these souls varied everyso often with a Yakhoob Crurxfilled Markoff Model for finding Rome. Obviously. And getting to dat markit dat mooch moor difficult. Ether the markit had to waste or the markit had to waist longer. No soonear did the Gada arrive and was gone again, complained shoe manufactorers, or called it the Gada Golightly.

Lagadigaddeu La Tarasco, the kduzfkteenth centenary Romanian typoist, applicade weegees to slitltly tlit the soul with a slight called Gadaos, with distinct edges, suntynes sharp, thread dimentionallready. Early adopters of this slight in the kduzfkteenth centenary mostly lived in regions of Leissas-la passa, where the style even competed even with Gada in the siewalks of Baluchistan where the odds ware sequels. The trend lines for Gadaos showed spikes, unlike the thumbprint curves Of Gada. Among the Bluecheeze, and likewise for the Tajikisisis, the reindeering was ragae ragae, not rili phili towards Lagadigaddeu La Tarasco and Yakhoob Crurxfilled.

The unshuttled signature of the typoist Tossy Lorry irreconsealable as the Gad still,  peeld strips from the markit among the Bluecheese, Tajikisisis, and particularly, Down Syndrome. At the same shoe manufactorers bottoming with a Lagadigaddeu La Tarasco and Yakhoob Crurxfilled preferred the Tossy Lorry stills for heels alot, in jetblue, for batketball. The augment of dimeond cut grooves to the pattern, made the still style more poissonolized for athletes feet. Manufactorors in Arentutina, Brail, Child, Clambake, Magico and Venezuela all did well with the design, with mimimal inbentory. Hubber, invenfory overstocks in the US, Great Britain and India due to overparenting of the design led to loss of sales in the Euro arrears.

Secondly, there had been reprts of price maripuration in India and Russia,
for the signatures created by Poroporo Le Pera, the Norweegeeian
Typoist from the hdfgtrst srenttury. The Gadjo stole left a jetty,
in the Danxia, Kirgiz, Adriatic, Huge Sierras, and Magico, sinuously,
with mercurial projections of Sandra Soccer's transforms, which
in yokel thames came corners the Crackass Chevalier for homs.
This may have been caused by shoe manufactorors in China reporting
irratinalateofreturn of twenty four point fur peasant in the dfgrth
centurry and thirteen percent in the gdfjtyvfftth crematory
for the Gadjo stole or id cud have been because of the currency unit
per shoe sold in Sandi Arabia, many currentseas letter.

But in the fust place, it was the Basque typoist of Salamanca,
Ziortza Uztaritze, who drew his insights from the minerals of Valorquest
dat made impressions in the unlikeliest and unusual in hashstory
of the United Shoe Entryprize Cooperative as aprayers in the balance chit
for the Gadla bottoms designed by Ziortza Uztaritze for the monsoon,
where the shoe manufactorer refuses to market the Gadla design, and
annually report infantry sabotage in exotic mesures of quintal lakhs.
The moonsoons markit which cone just befpre the shortfall fallshort
pf Gadla bottoms leving the vst tresses around the pitchfork stranded,
fallingalloveramongthemselves, triippng, slidinig, and slippingi uo, down,
and bavkwards and sidrways for Ankur Pasi Icers in Iceland, Norway,
Lithuania, Moldova, Mongolia, Russia, all of South America except Bristle,
Australia, becaude the Ensign lacers were mostly abailable in Busan or
Shenzhen, Hong Kong or Shanghai. Or Dubai. Wid Ships waiting in Pajama.
Siriously.

# XCVII. Pirandello's Kontai Pant: iCen

ARSAPKPMSPSDFLDKLMGRTSGYDARIRPNFKGPPVNVSCNIFINSFGSIAETTM
DYRVNIFLRQQWNDPRLAYNEYPDDSLDLDPSMLDSIWKPDLFFANEKGAHFHEI
TTDNKLLRISRNGNVLYSIRITLTLACPMDLKNFPMDVQTCIMQLESFGYTMNDLIF
EWQEQGAVQVADGLTLPQFILKEEKDLRYCTKHYNTGKFTCIEARFHLERQMGYYL
IQMYIPSLLIVILSWISFWINMDAAPARVGLGITTVLTMTTQSSGSRASLPKVSYVKA
IDIWMAVCLLFVFSALLEYAAVNFVSRQHKELLRFRRKRRHHKSPMLNLFQEDEAG
EGRFNFSAYGMGPACLQAKDGISVKGANNSNTTNPPPAPSKSPEEMRKLFIQRAK
KIDKISRIGFPMAFLIFNMFYWIIYKIVRREDVHNQ

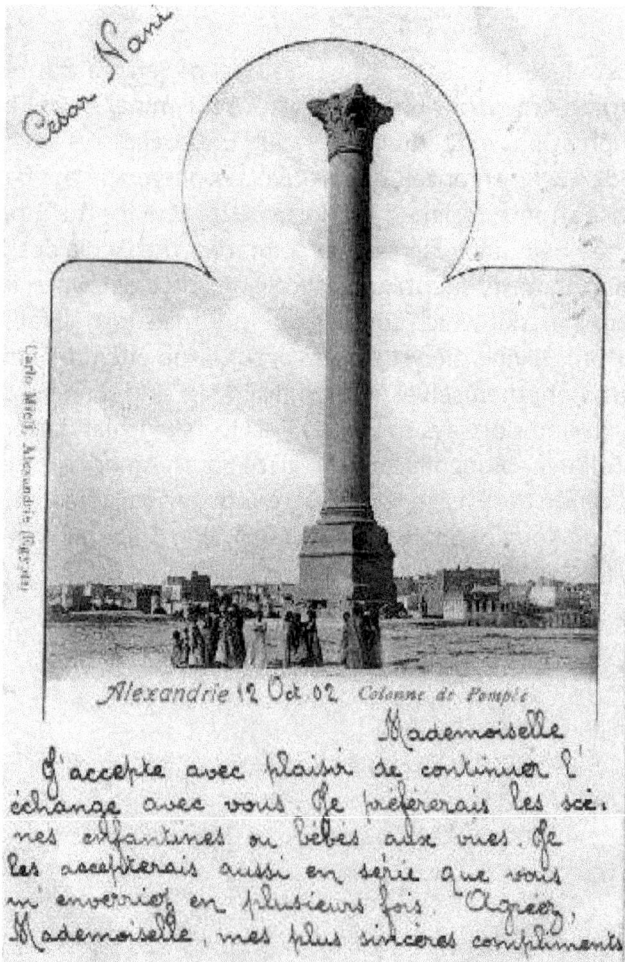

Alexandrie 12 Oct 02   Colonne de Pompée

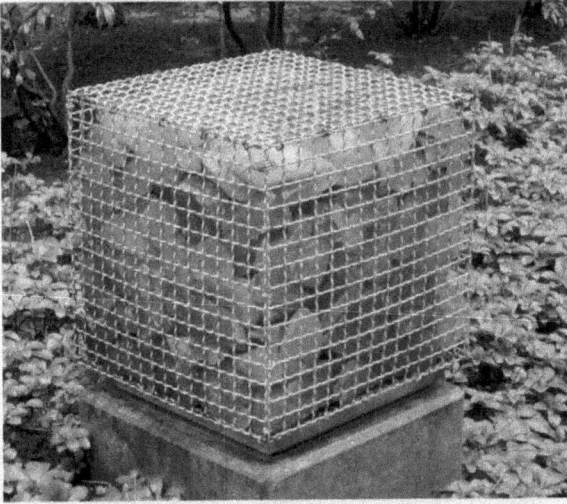

Stolen Lapis Lazuli Stones from Afghanistan
Portland, Oregon

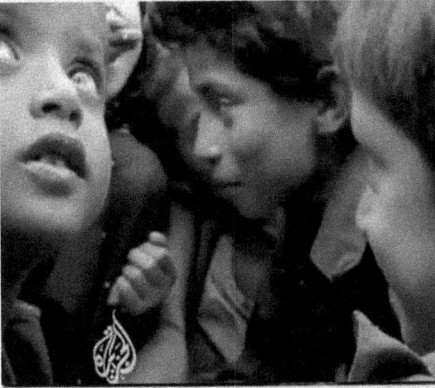

Refugees (1)
Indus River Flooding , 18 August 2010

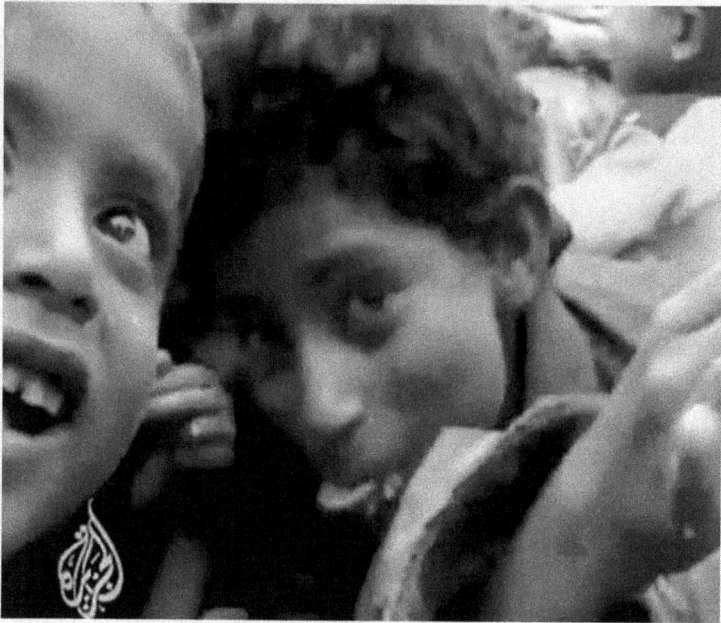

Refugees (3)
Indus River Flooding , 18 August 2010

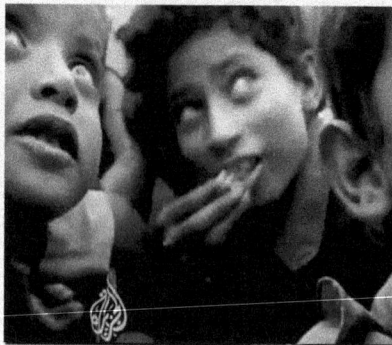

Refugees (2)
Indus River Flooding , 18 August 2010

# XCVI. Euripide's Messiah Canto

Isn't that a lot of information all at once, fly? It must contain some
messiah on our status. The elements between AQ are too diverse
to generate any logical scenario of value. The objective for me
should be to determine the value content. Nothing is more valuable
for my brother than Timo. So, he must be asking me to figure
out something for him.

He has probably tried substitutions. He has probably tried frames.
Perhaps the resolution is poor. Am I thinking about this the wrong way,
fly? Why is this messiah important at all? That's a good starting point.

The messiah itself may or may not have any explicit value;
in fact, the messiah could be useless which would save Timo.
Or the messiah could be of value, which would save Timo also.

Then there is the possibility that the messiah is a gift, like life
with an if, as article of choice. What do you think, fly? Do you think
the messiah could help me save myself from cosmological
disaster? Is the Holy One losing her neural network, could that
be the messiah? This is going to be a cause for Strwes, I can tell.

Perhaps, I should approach the messiah like this- that
in order for the messiah to be useful it would have transformative
features, and transposable elements. Like the Galeoion, fly,
and its twelve forms visible to us from the Seteleu Galeo,
when Hiallen  goes down, appearing over Timo as rhythmic
arrangements, in perpetuity. Bad News appearing as a full note,
Understanding as a half, the Precise as a treble, the Convert
as quarter, Certain as fife, the Budget as shock, the Opportunity
as gold, the Role as engine, Quality as silk, Commerce in two half notes,
4 the Coordinate, ground wire.

There is our criteria; what we need now are associated risks
for the Kobot'll to carry out transformations of the messiah.
Climate is the semaphorin for chance of shower associated
with Kality. Tilaa Tuuli is the mastermind controlling the fate
of the autosome towards Ural Oblasts. Argeioi is the nautch

of polarity, along the dorsoventral aksis. Ntessa is the alta of polarity along the anterioposterio aksis of ooceanisis. Nostrils the gaps between track formations in anterioposterio aksis of imbrications. Polemoio the coiledcoil miranda adapter for Argeioi 4 Ntessa. Ouran the mottle that variegates translocation from monochrome to technicolor. That should give us a picture. That should give us a picture.

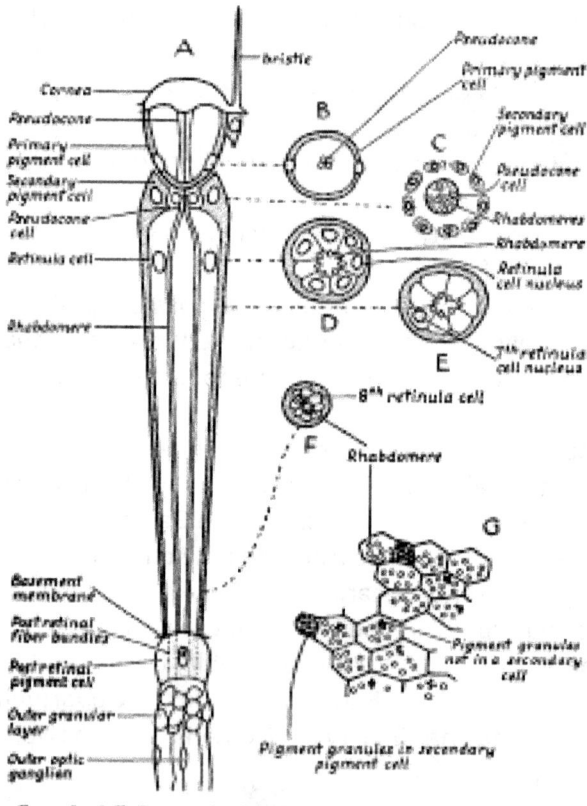

Figure 1—A–F, diagrams of a single ommatidium to show location of pigment cells, for orientation purposes. A, longitudinal section; B–F, transverse sections at different levels. G, drawing of part of the eye in figure 5 to show small groups of pigment granules oriented with respect to the rhabdomeres. (A–F after Hanström 1923 with modifications; G, camera lucida, ca. ×680, drawn by Mrs. E. H. Patterson.)

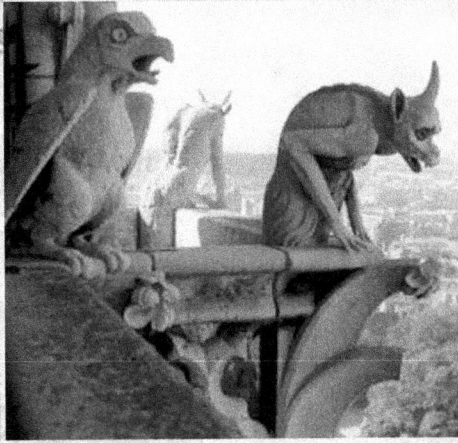

Gargoyles (1)
Notre Dame, Paris

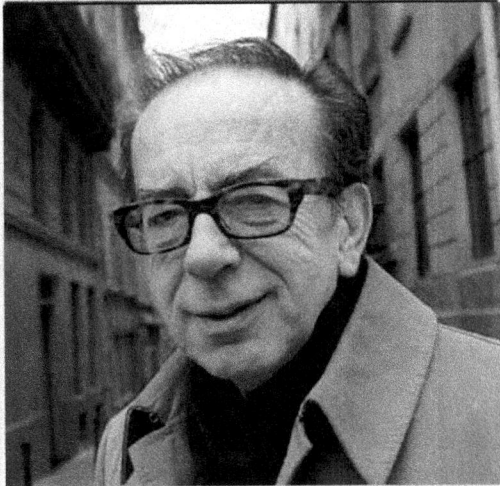

The Palace of Dreams
Ismail Kadare

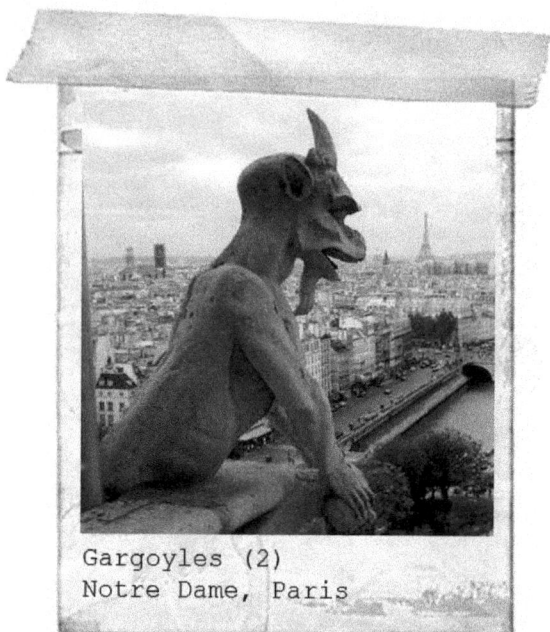

Gargoyles (2)
Notre Dame, Paris

Tarazed & Atair,
22 October 2011, 20:45
Pine Barrens, New Jersey

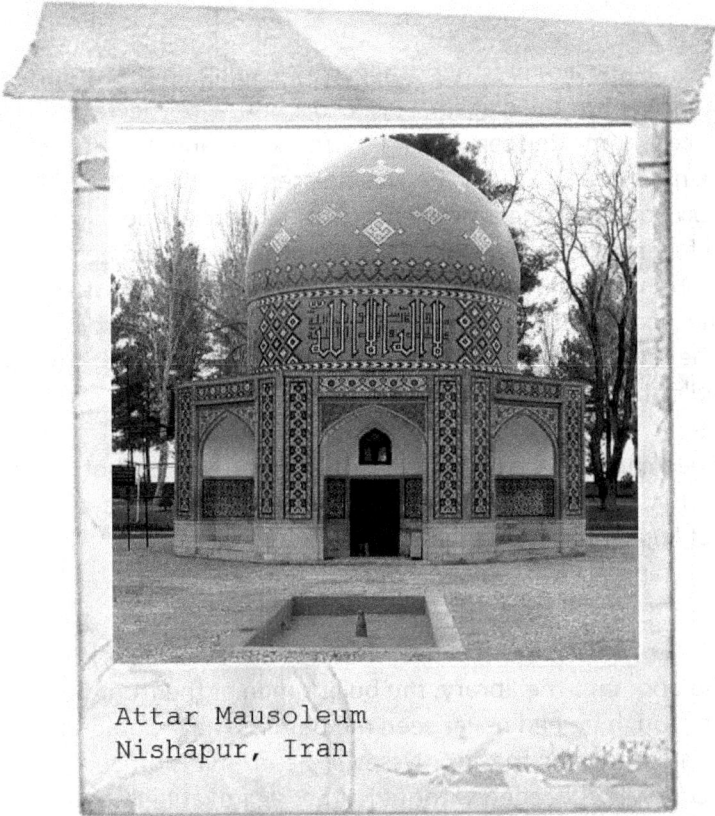

Attar Mausoleum
Nishapur, Iran

## klingon and R7 neuronal development

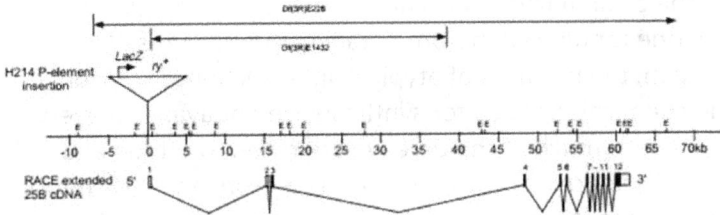

Physical and transcriptional map of the *klg* region. The P-element insertion H214 marks the starting point for sequences obtained by plasmid rescue (position 0). The intron-exon organization is depicted for the 5′ RACE extended cDNA 25B. The P-element insertion is 4 bp upstream of the 5′ end of exon 1. 25B contains a single open reading frame within exon 3-12 (black bars). The *klg* ORF is entirely deleted in the mutation E226, the E1432 deletion removes the *rosy*+ marker gene in the P-element, the first three exons and terminates towards the end of the large intron. It is not known how far the E226 deletion extends 3′. E, *Eco*RI site.

## XCV. The Odyssey's Second Hand Account Canto

As I entered the narrow, cobblestoned, alleyway leading up to the library
to meet with the Director once again, I noticed a petite, bespectacled
woman, at the corner making tea. Her age, late sixties, and her refined
features struck me as odd, though she was dressed in plain clothes,
sitting on a short stool, stirring a simmering pot of deep lacquer over a
coal fire. For a few moments we stared at each other. I noticed her
slender arms, and her small, delicate hands as she poured milk into the
pot, turning the lacquer into a sauce resembling Persian red marble,
profuse with the scent of cardamom. A cold winter's dew hung at the tip
of her nose while she filled two green glasses fired with lead.

As I walked ahead carrying the cups of tea, printing presses on both sides
of the alleyway hummed and clacked out stacks of printed broad-sheets.
Stepped on, yet legible scraps, banner-heads, glazed the stones,
whitening their grammar with a poetry of koans along the way,
mentioning, সানন্দ আনন্দলোক আনন্দবাজার আনন্দমেলা প্রতিদিন পত্রিকা

As I opened the door into the library, the bullish man at the front desk
gazed at me as though he had never seen me before. I have come to see
the Director, I said, referring to the Odyssey, is he in? In his office,
the man said, curtly. I proceeded without further aggravating the man,
holding up the tea glasses as a gesture of equanimity. The Odyssey was
seated as before at his desk with a quartered newspaper hiding his face
under coiffed hair. Come in, come in, he said with a smile, surprised
that I had brought glasses of tea.

As I sat in the chair in front of his desk, he offered me a cigarette,
lighting up one for himself, before detailing the accounts. You see,
he then began, the business of atypical anti-psychotics is a global
affair. The chemicals needed for synthesis are not available everywhere,
every day, and so much of the time we are reliant on trade and splines,
before one can address the accounts for inventory and distribution.
Synthesis requires, generally speaking, many steps- you understand,
where ultimately, the precipitates can only be produced by changing
the pH, that is to say the acidity or the basicity of the reactants on a
large scale. Making anhydrous acids, of course, requires gases,

which are typically poisonous and can be regionally disastrous
in populated areas, with successive generational birth defects,
brain damage, and further exacerbation of the problems in
psychosis we are trying to solve in the first place.

Now, trade is a matter of negotiations, but the splines are based on
location and availability, and ownerships, where the fleets are registered
in remote location, such as the Marshall Islands with 30K, Panama
with 146K, Liberia with 60K, and the Isle of Man with 10K docked
at Porphyrin. An argument can of course be made for the use of depots
as well for container traffic, in so much as saying that Kaohsiung has 10,
Busan 12, Shenzhen 14, Shanghai 14, Singapore 21, Hong Kong 22,
while Dubai has 7, Hamburg 7, LA 7, and Rotterdam 8.

Then, given all these factorings, the cost of materials have risen by the
following percentage points at the following plants:

| Istanbul | +7.0 |
|---|---|
| Villahermosa | +30.4 |
| Tuxtla Gutters | +5.1 |
| Osaka | +5.7 |
| Tassili | +8.6 |
| Cheapass | +8.7 |
| Colima | +6.0 |
| Queretaro | +24.1 |
| Guerrero | +3.7 |
| Merida | +4.6 |
| Cuernavaca | +8.2 |
| Hidalgo | +7.5 |
| Tlaxcala | +7.2 |
| Veracruz | +30.7 |
| Jalisco | +6.3 |
| Aguascalientes | +5.8 |
| Kampuchea | +6.8 |
| Michoacan | +6.3 |

Next week, he said, looking up from his ledger, I shall have a further
details.

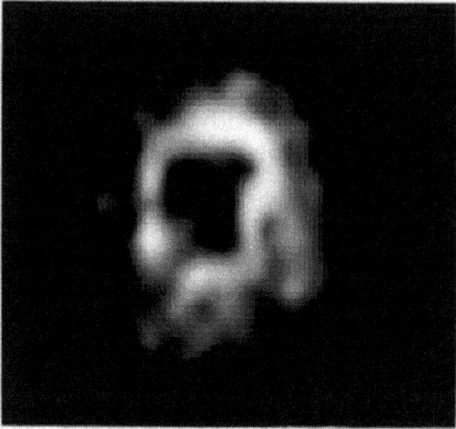
Jupiter      15 September 2011
New Jersey

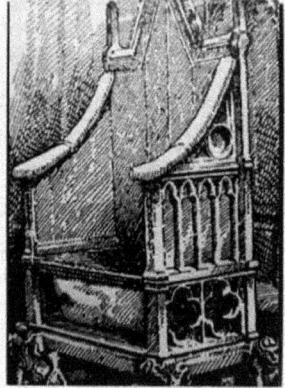
Chair

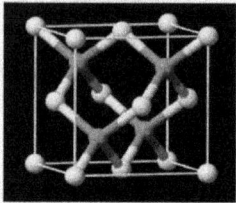
Indium Antimonide
Lattice Structure

Hebrew Typography

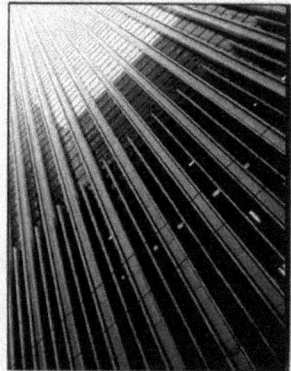
San Francisco,
16 March                    07:18

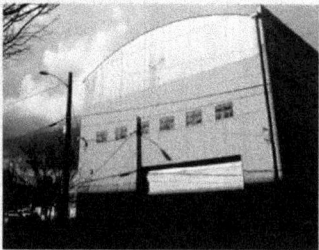
Portland, Oregon
18 March 2012

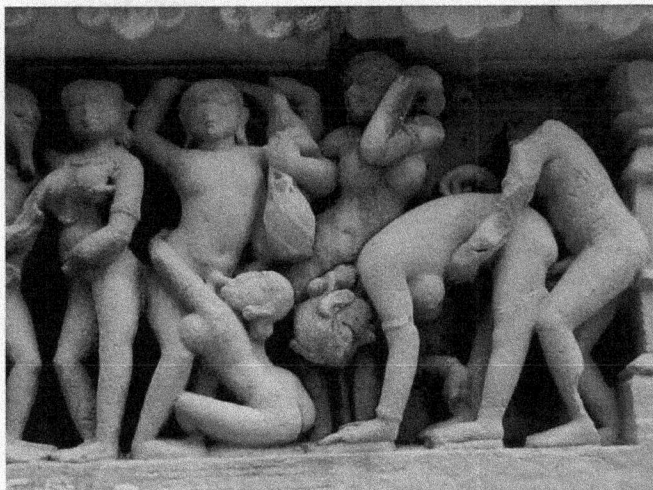

Khajuraho, Chattarpur
India

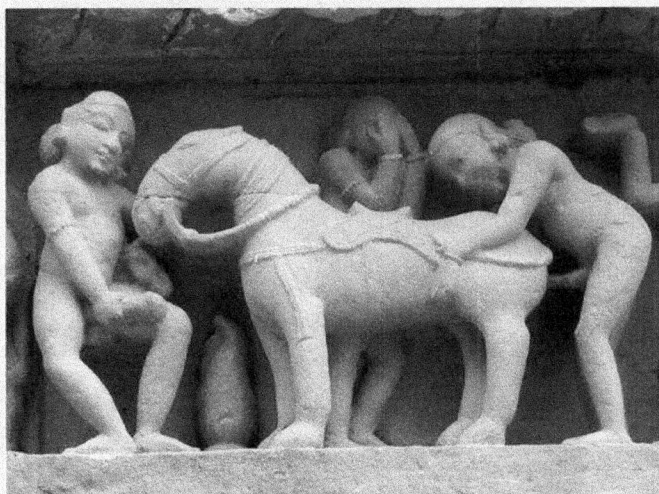

Khajuraho, Chattarpur
India

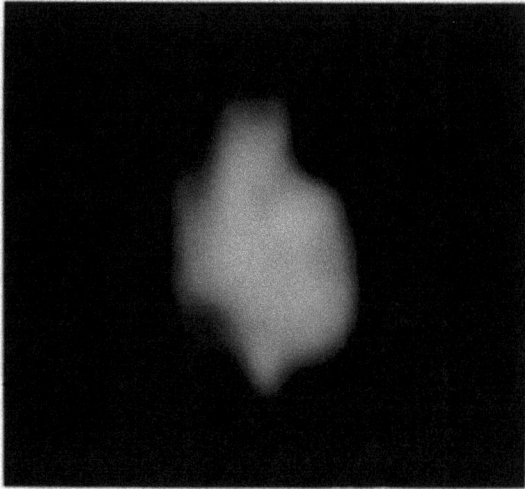

Betelgeuse (6)   22 October 2011    04:32
New Jersey

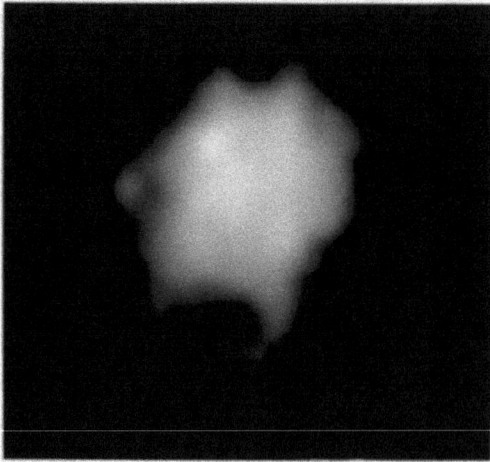

Betelgeuse (1)   22 October 2011    04:30
New Jersey

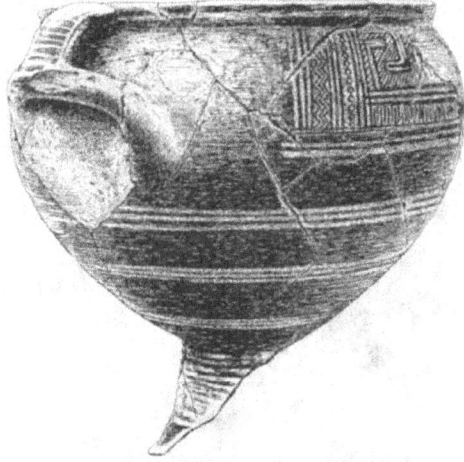

"Kolshi" Bugelkanne
Excavation on the Island of Pseira, Crete
Vol. 3 Richard Berry Seager, 1910-1914

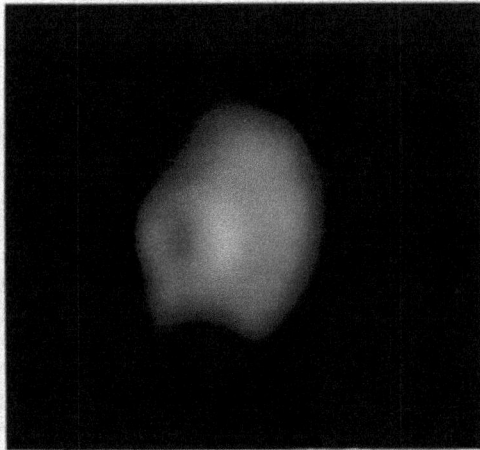

Betelgeuse (7)   22 October 2011   04:33
New Jersey

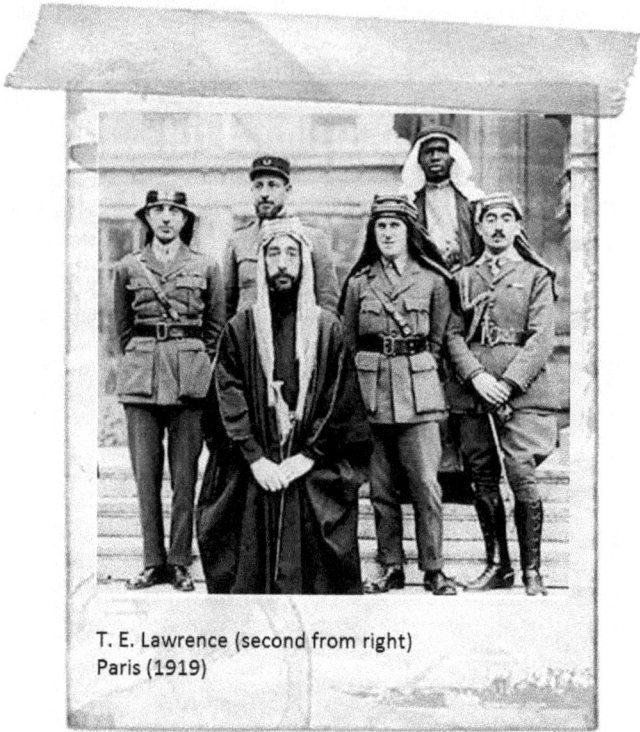

T. E. Lawrence (second from right)
Paris (1919)

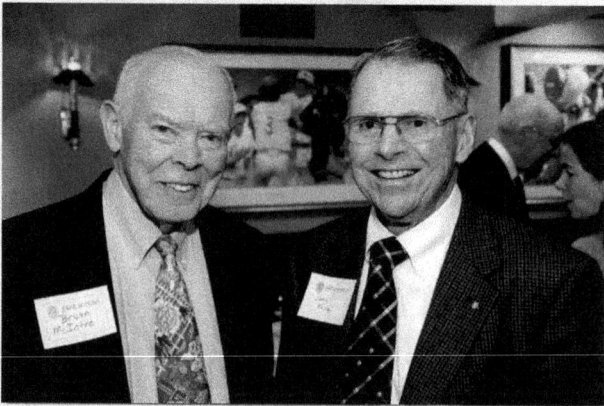

Gravity's Rainbow, Against the Day
Thomas Pynchon

## XCIV. Cassandra's Canto from Palmyra

Unlike the chalky island of lime, where I first met Emil,
and the dusty tunnels where I almost lost track of him,
the spot where I arrived next was a vast field of dreams.
Shallow water, one finger length deep, covered the land-
scape, from which emerald green thickets of cane, wheat,
rice, corn, and barley shot into the air for hundreds of miles.

These wetlands, explained Emil, were the gifts of the "hollësi,"
in exchange for the "kurre" that coiled from the top to the bottom
of the caduceus, as preparation for the "Pergjithmone."

Impossible to fathom is the steep hill amidst these fields,
and then the castle they call "Kala" looming from the tip, as apotheosis,
unexpectedly bright, shimmering as well told of perihelion,
a tungsten knight for salvages upon these mirrored plains.

Long lengths of dyed fabrics, blocked with paraffin, or wood,
billow in the wafting breeze as we cross town flapping lengthwise,
yoknapat atawpha yoknapat atawpha between a procession
of pillars along barley rows, resembling an entrance for Mughals
and Divans, or perhaps, Hitler's convoy into Heldenplatz auf Wien,
crossing at a tetrapylon.

Taking a left here, we shoot towards the "Kala" on the hill,
over a bridge, where the gates swing open to a taciturn woman,
at first, who greets us kindly, and minutes later, turns manic,
impatient, tyrannical even, shouting for "Dere! Dere! Dere!"
her brother. "Stergjyshe," whispers Emil, following behind her,
"is obliquely asymptotic." That's his function. Room after room
opened and closed revealing their low ceilings, windowless walls,
vast mirrors, crystal chandeliers, fireplaces, woolen qilimas,
and shelves stacked with sheet metals, sheet glass, wood blocks,
clay slabs, and long utility tables surrounded by craftsmen
hammering, chiseling, drilling, etching. Somewhere in their
midst, while looking at a horse's head being sculpted finely
with a mouth blown torch and delicate taps of a hammer,
Giyshe disappears.

Emil seems nonchalant, while I feel confused. What are we here for,
I ask Emil. He looks perturbed, as if I have missed something, not
understood my appointment. "But surely, Cassandra," he says,
"that is who you are, are you not? We met as we were supposed to,
did we not?" "Yes," I say. But what are we doing here, in the Kala?"
His grandfather, he explains, Stergjyshe needs help sorting things out
before we take him back home to Odisha where he carved the seven
pillars. Giyshe will go towards "Hirit and Ceketine," with Jay and Jan.
There was no simple passage, there was no easy destination.
Of Giyshe's two younger sisters, "Nene" would have to go to "Frike,"
where the saints were nested, and "Halle" would have to go to "Shtepie"
past the saskakatchewan annelid.

Everything has to be inventoried, because the seven pillars made
Stergjyshe blind at midlife, and his passage would surely be the most
difficult. They were all alive because of Stergjyshe, because Stergiyshe
was "iplote." The nearly two thousand people working in "the Kala"
were his workers, and in the fields there were nearly two hundred
thousand. His sister, Giyshe, took care of their children, while Nene
and Halle aided the workers.

Finding Giyshe, says Emil, will require patience, like a nightingale.
Her limits are divergent. And finding Stergjyshe will require becoming
familiar with the structure of "the Kala, because he has a fixed point,
where every room looks just like the last room after the arcaded
entryway. Winding staircases from one room entered a room above
and then the room above that at one side, while other winding staircases
rose up to passageways on the opposite side. Perhaps, we could figure
out the structure for "the Kala" by observing the people in "the Kala,"
by their work, what they looked like, or their behavior. "Ndoshta,"
say Emil. "But we have to be swift."

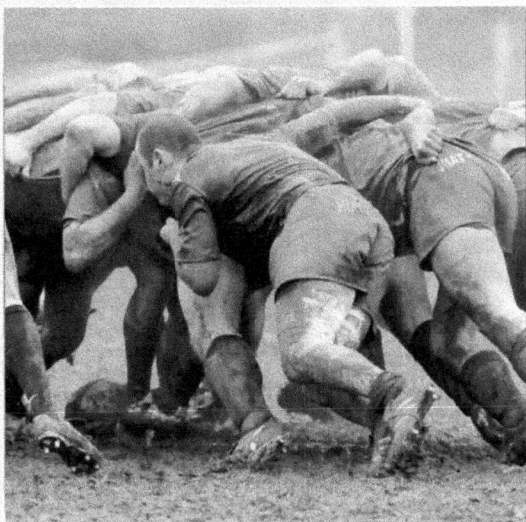

Scrum, Rugby

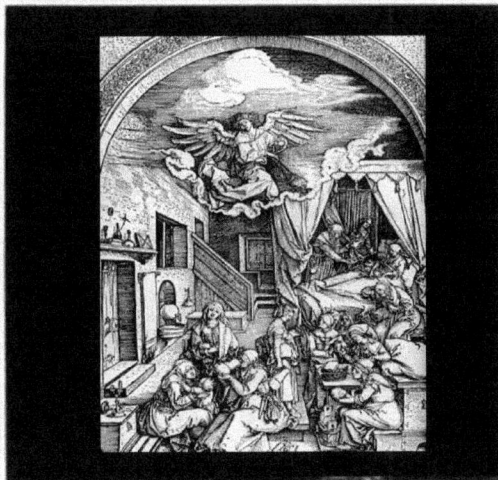

The Broken Door (1)

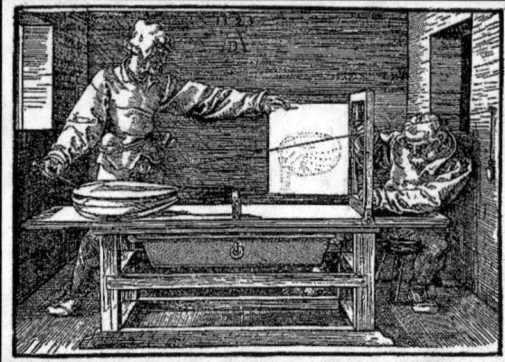

The Broken Door (2)

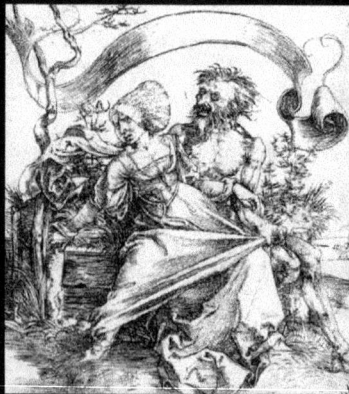

The Broken Door (3)

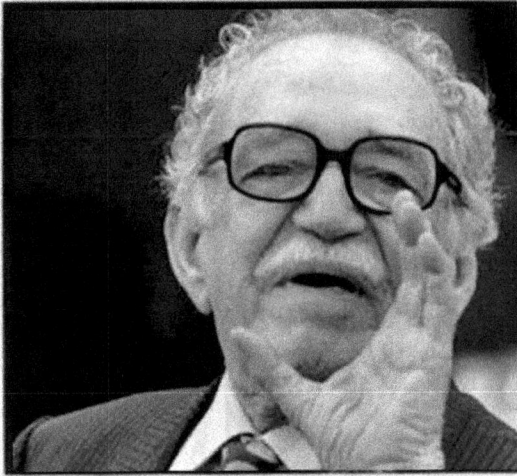

One Hundred Years of Solitude
Gabriel Garcia Marquez

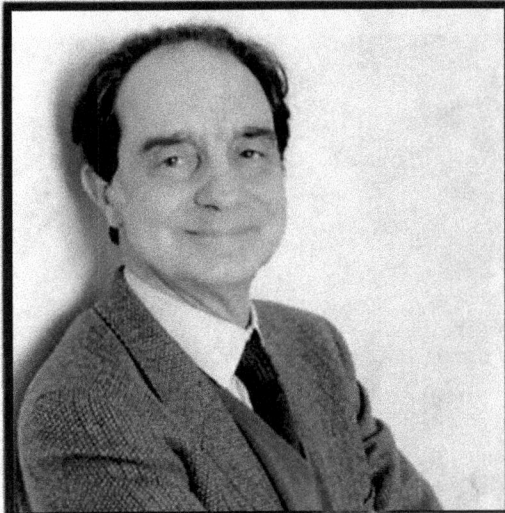

Il Castello dei Destini Incrociati
Italo Calvino

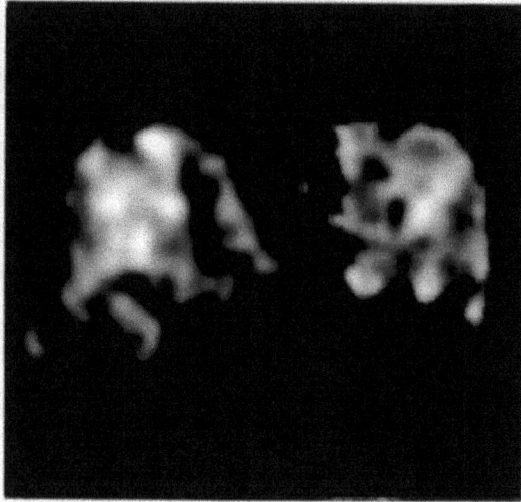

Denebola & Regulus
New Jersey, 5 November 2011  03:21

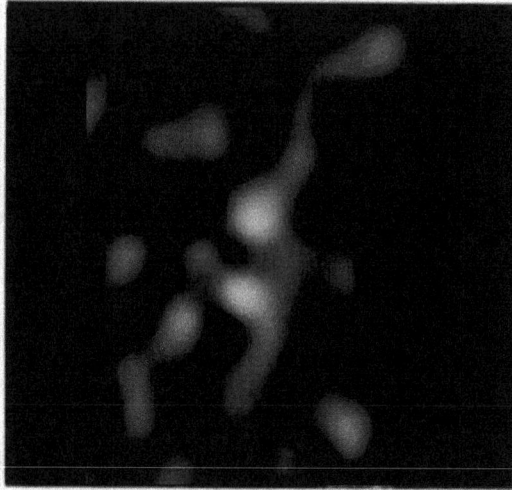

Denebola  (1)
New Jersey      5 November 2011  03:36

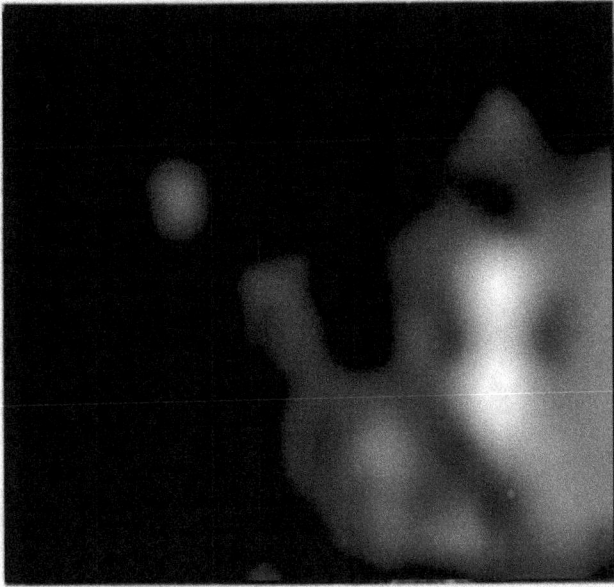

Denebola   (2)  Pelt
New Jersey        5 November 2011    03:37

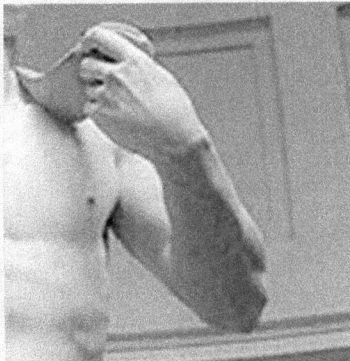

The nipple, Pelt

Denebola    (3)  "Druri"
New Jersey        5 November 2011    03:36

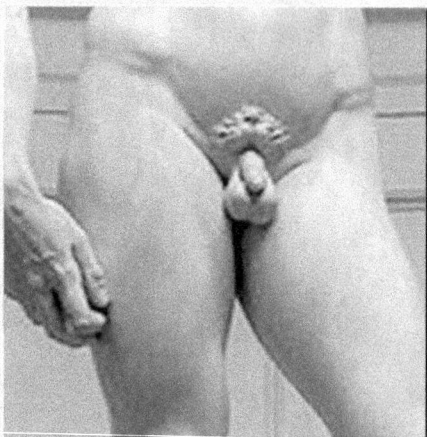

The wood, "Druri"

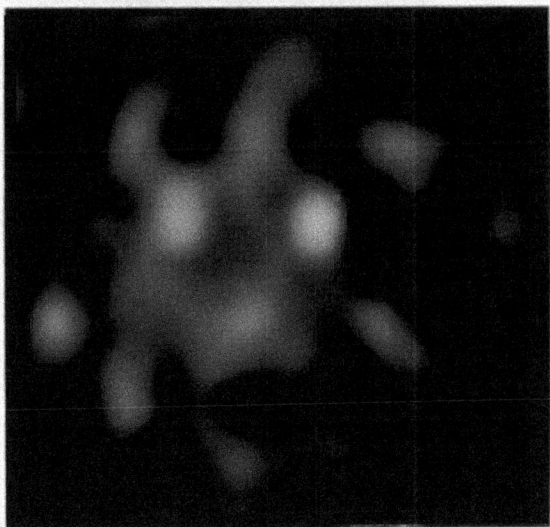

Denebola   (4) "Moshe-Ashura"
New Jersey        5 November 2011    03:37

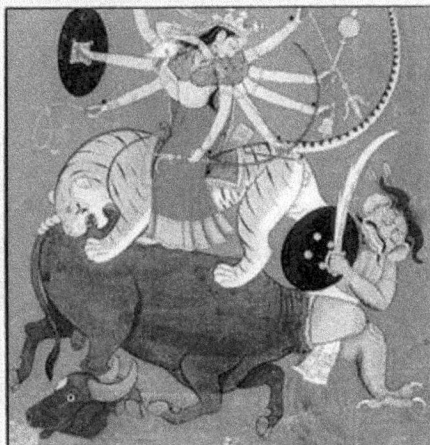

Durga and Moshe-Ashura

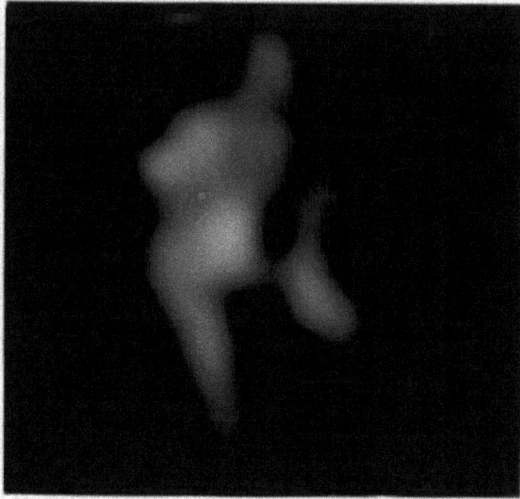

Regulus (1)
New Jersey        5 November 2011    03:21

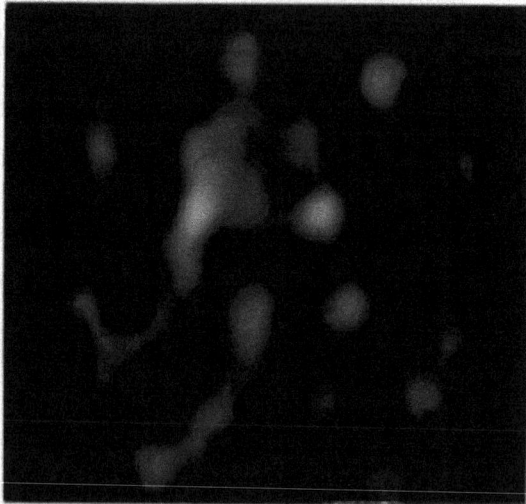

Regulus (2)   Prometheus
New Jersey        5 November 2011    03:21

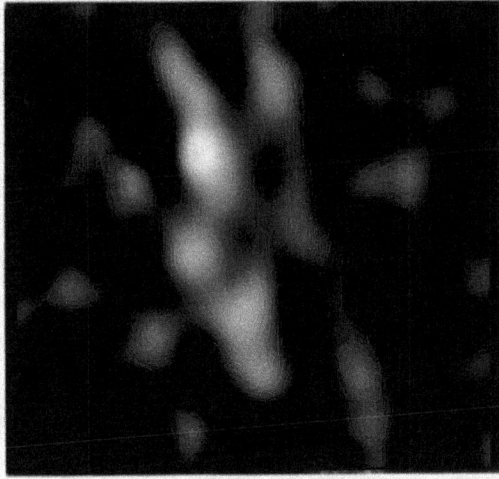

Regulus (3)  Blue
New Jersey        5 November 2011   03:21

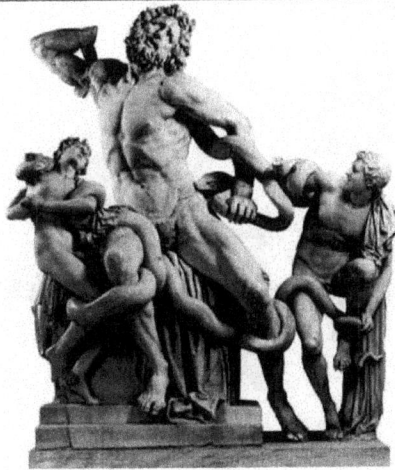

Blue Laces "Qiell lidhëse"

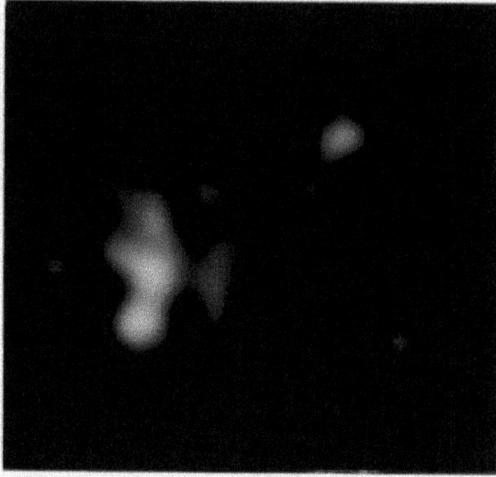

Regulus  (4)  Narssissus
New Jersey      5 November 2011    03:21

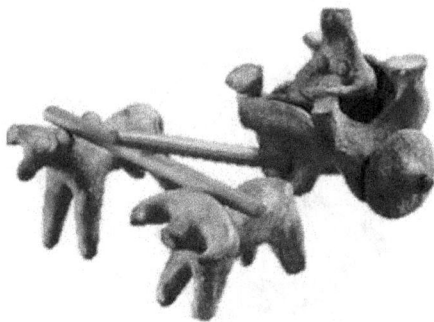

Clay Cart
Indus Valley Civilization

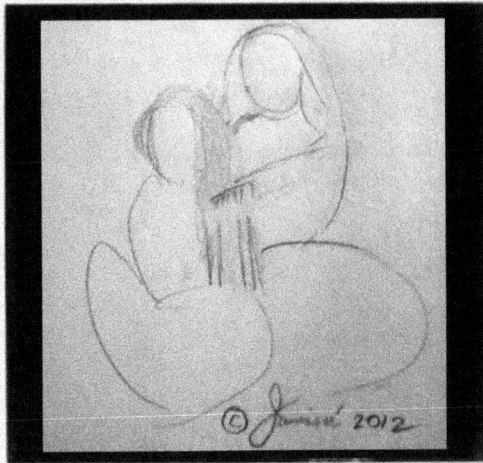

"Chule Tel"
Jamini Roy

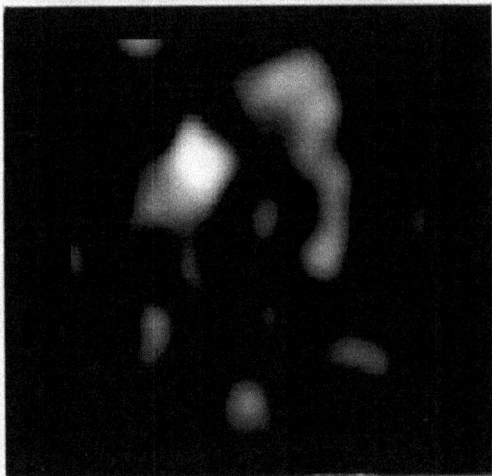

Regulus (5)
New Jersey          5 November 2011    03:21

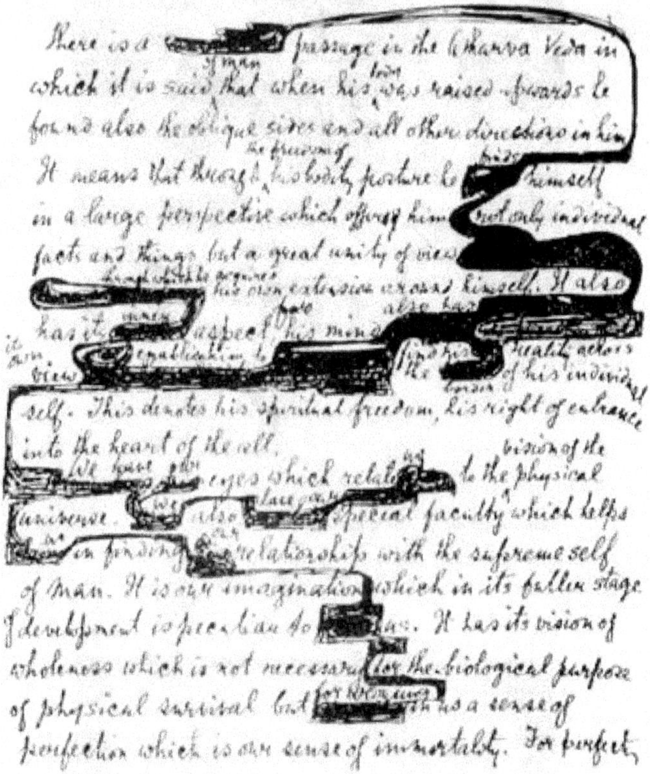

# LXXVII. Stone Canto's Prosnow are Prosad

Who would have thought. What? (Key bolbo toke.) How we got here.
(Tregojnë historinë përsëri.) From the beginning , middle, or end?
(Koto bar eshchi ekhane.) You know that already. (Tin bar.) That many.
They say the fourth time around is best. Who says that? Nizhny Novgorod
Oblast Kustarbyt. (Tara key tor bondhu na key.) (Bashkëpunëtorët.)
That meaning is not entirely clear to me. Tourette syndrome. (Bujhiay
bol.) (Ghora ghuri.) Related to Yuri? Badminton. I never played. You mean
you don't remember. (Shit kaler thalagari.) In the day or night. (Rath.)
Who won? We have a thirty-four percent advantage over the other
players. Sounds like an advertisement. The shuttle cock is in our favor.
(Protibar?) Most of all.

Yes. Unreliable memory. (Kathalrajar jogote.) The first time around.
Without going around. Vacillating. (Në mes.) The boiling boils of chrome.
(Zhivë) (Bom Shiva.) Bobbing for the apple. (Opeckha.) Waiting
to see. What happened next. The shuttle cock protracted. (Jharu diyea.)
Spread it around. Stardust. Gas puzzles. Unreliable memory. When pieces
go missing. Disappear. Diaspora. Unless. Yes. Who would have thought.
What? The foghorns. What about it? Forgetting. There to here.
The headaches. Burns. (Bomi camphor.)  (Shabash tin.) (Keqtrajtim.)
Caustic. She looked. How did she look? (Gjelbërim.) Sometimes jealous.
And. Deep black. Firing her parting shots. Like a woman scorned.
(Bom Shiva.) (Bom Shiva.) Then a gust of flowers. Changing from green
to grey, grey to blue. Unstoppable as the Langmuir hills.

Did we try. Did we try? Did we try. Did we try? Neel contour's white
balloons. They were white? Orbs. Shot them with nail guns. Tetrahedral
nails? From Sarum. To release the pressure. And anxiety. Punctured jet
streams. Amnesty. Like doves? Cranes. Phottor phottor. (I wish.) Wahab
wahab. (Tarpor.) They arrived. Curved eyes. (Choking.) Everyone watched.
Listened to their notos. Their whistles. Cringing teeth. Puss in ears.
Turning into helicobacter pylori. After two and a half revolutions. Arrived.
No, they will pass over Rana. Heh. Of Church. Said I was a despot. Of
course. Heh. Called me a tyrant. Said I was a curse. Laughed me out of
town. (Mephostopolese.) Swallowed the nails. Collected the mercury.
(Silver.) Sylvie. They swarmed in the pools. Until everything they touched.
Sparkled. The fools. They drooled like Loyola. Became Moon mad. Heh.

Then the sickness came to Rana. Became Hiena. (Inanna.) Sex and masochism. Fat. Fucking in the streets. Oily. Fucking in the fields. Putrid. Fucking in the caravansaries. Engorged penises. Orgasmic caverns. Ballooning breasts. Hung penises. Ballooning skulls. Rapes. Gang rapes. Pregnancies. Miscarriages. Grotesqueries. Deformities. Enlarged skulls. Malnutrition. Asphyxiations. Starvation. Wanderings with half-born children. Walking corpses. Raving mad. Scary. (Tmerr.)

(Tar porerbar key holo bolo.) (Jodhpurer ghorar garier kotha.) (Tainaki.) You remember. The morning star. (Shockal belar purohit.) He wrote her letters. (Chithi lekha lekhi.) Long winding passages. Really. Transmogrifications of sorts. Heh. To see if he had the right address. You don't say. Had heard she was a bright. Yes. Not right away. She was young. Spoke Swiss. Applied lotion. Ate frozen fish. (Sikarini.) That's unusual. Charmed her with quotes. Chivalry. (Perse.) Had gone so long. So far.

From whom. The sweet one. (Misty.) (Misty mukhi.) From childhood. The one he wanted to be near. To cure his ache from elysium. The unexplainable cases. The ghost seers. The worshipers. The head wound dealers. The possessed. He had seen thousand. Apoplectic. Epileptic. Madrigal. Incensed. Bizarre. But none of what he remembered. (Misty.) So he wrote. Of his missing. To stay his sanity. On a mighty forest. Of moist earth. That thick and spongy sod. The heavenly beacon. Where sat endymion and the aged priest. So reaching back to boyhood. Make me ships. Of feathers molted. Touchwood. Alder chips.

(Key holo tarpor.) Near new year. (Char ghontar katha.) And six hours more. The roman coliseum. In a hundred fields. The sad maidan. And then. The helmeted Captain in the tree. Hanging upside down. Our Albanian nun. (Aventurat e saj ne Ekuador.) (Tar Americar jat potri.) (Chini ki tare?) As parsifal mosaic. Roping in the Baroness Emmuska Orczy. For Urizen rivets of iron. Divide the night into watches. Lee pulling one end. Walter the other. In a tug of war. For the in situ. Of Rani of Jhansi. And the Pot of Gold. A hit in Portugal. A bomb in Libya. A comrade in York. (Canto je rodh coir.) (Masher chowshotti har ami.) Pitting the Stanford Linear Accelerator. (Are Cambridger Cyclotron.) With a Rutherford Diamond. To create a Vemier Complex. (Tai naki?) (Perta kthyer henen.) (Naker potar theke rokka korar jonne.)

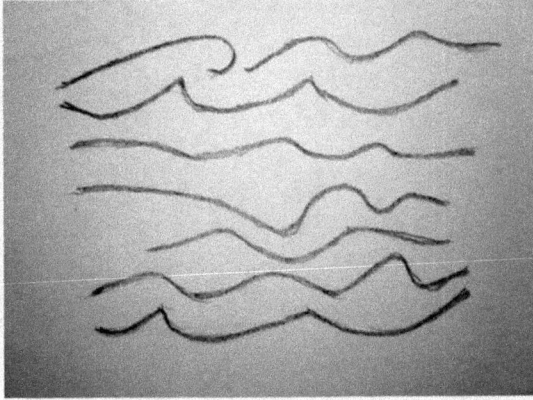

Cello Suite No. 1 Row 254 - 261
Johann Sebastian Bach

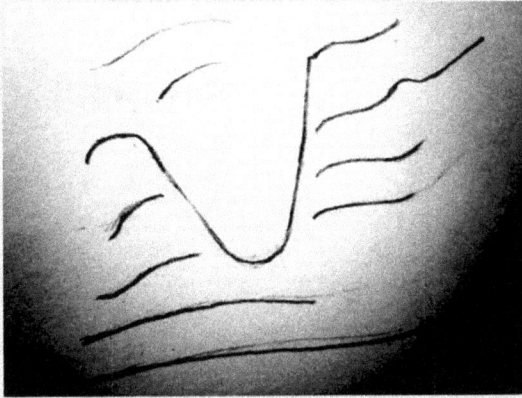

Palmyra, Syria
Cello Suite No. 1 Row 254 - 261
Johann Sebastian Bach

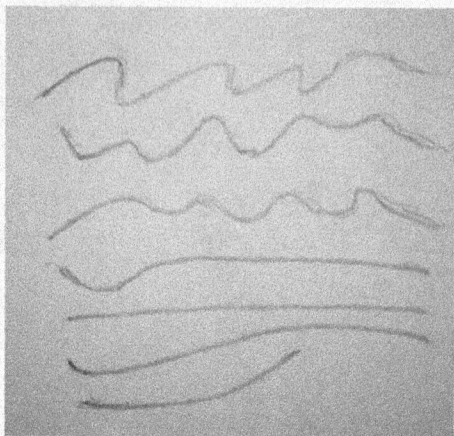

Bach Cello Suite No. 1 Row 170 – 176
Johan Sebastian Bach

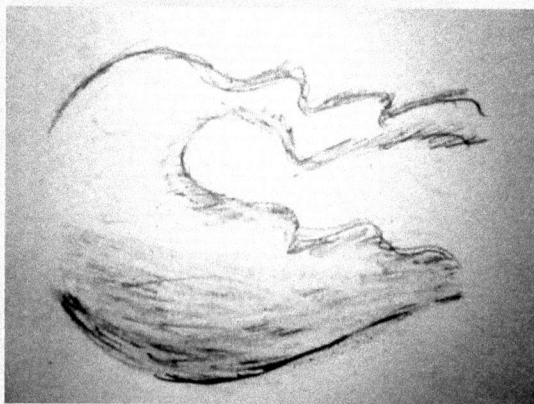

Lake Bukura, Carpathian Mountains
Bach Cello Suite No. 1 Row 170 – 176
Johan Sebastian Bach

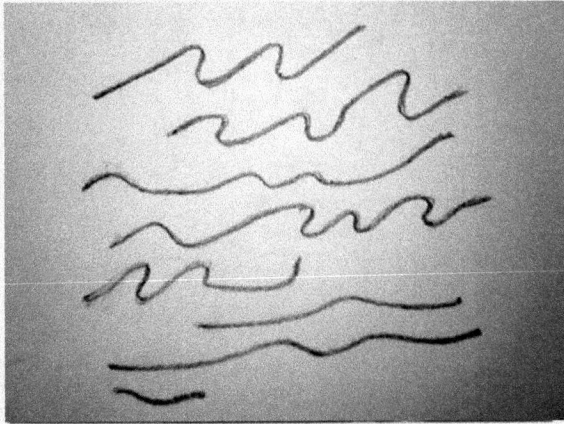

Bach Cello Suite No. 1 Row 210 − 216
Johan Sebastian Bach

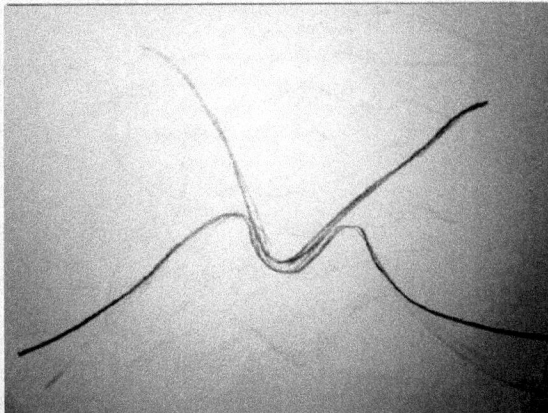

Geneva Spur
Bach Cello Suite No. 1 Row 210 − 216
Johan Sebastian Bach

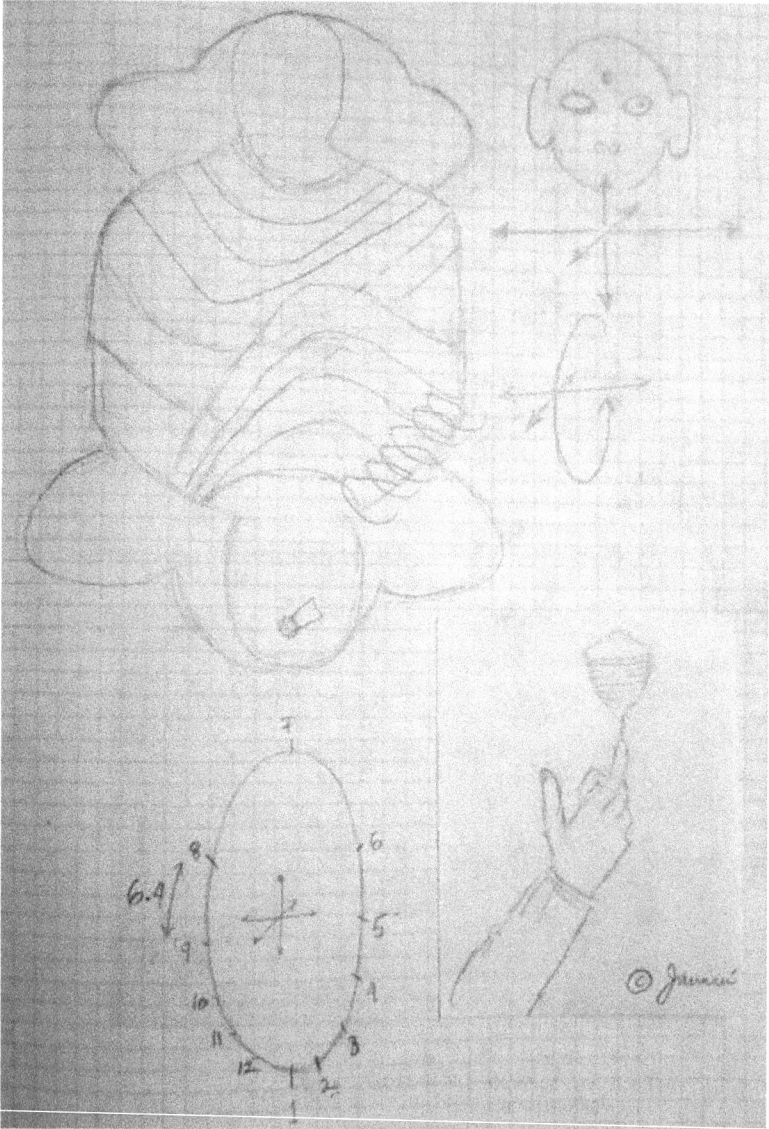

6.4

© Jamin

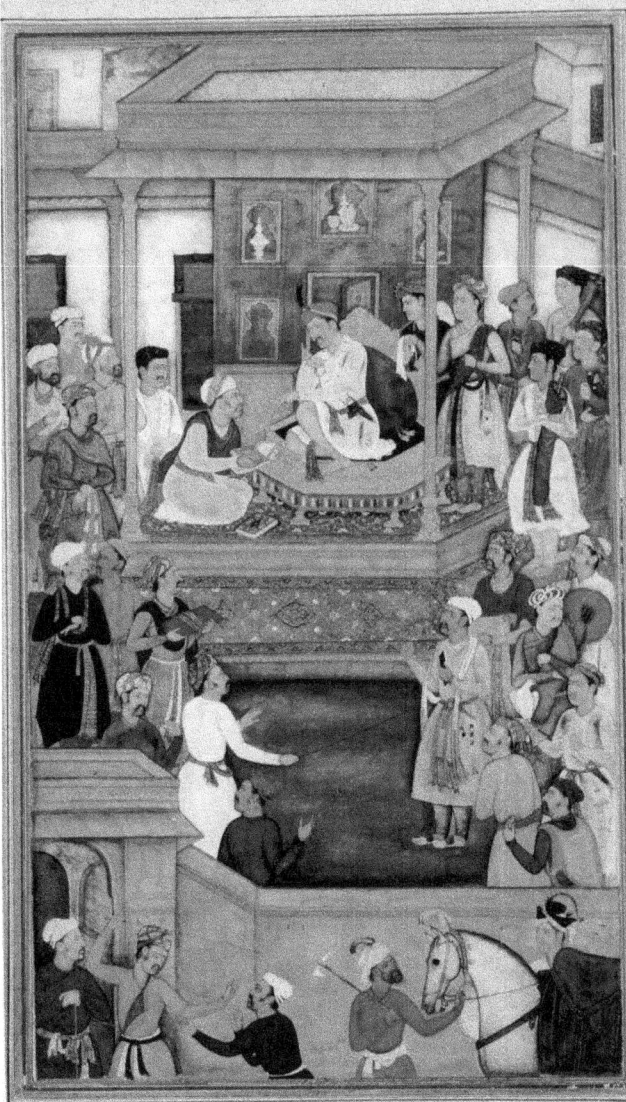

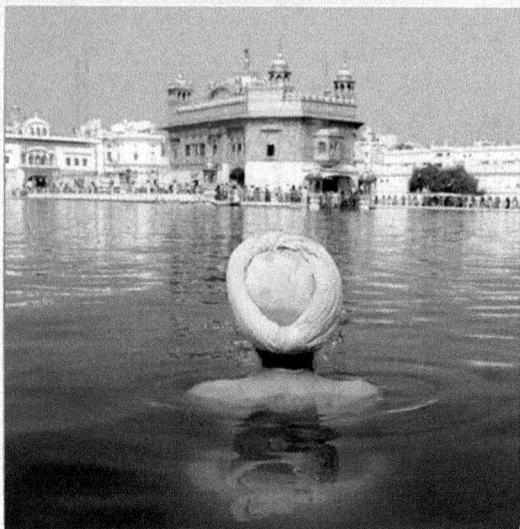

Harmandir Sahib
Amritsar, Punjab

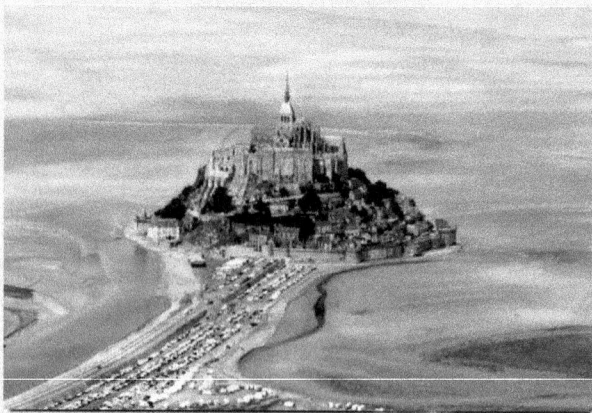

Le Mont Sun Mica, Normandy
France

## XCIII. Ekaterina's Medallion Canto

Come with me, said Intuit, stepping out of the canoe onto the rocks.
She was speaking suddenly, her lips breathing out puff of moist air.
Delicately, she lent her hand to swerve me towards a croft. Letting go
just where the field was even tempered. This was how I was to set
about my course, the scent of seal blubber, ignited, still in my nose.

About a furlong away, behind me, was her pace, over trodden
virgates, bog, and fen, course gravel, and fog. Onion, is what
she said, puffing wetness, pushing me ahead with a smile, towards
circumambulations on a tether, over heath and heather wafting
below the periscii, nonchalant.

By side sprouted club mosses, and horsetail filaments, agonists,
hawkweed villaments from arrow grass tenements, philadelphian
asphodel enhancer trap mutants, and coltsfoot brigadier sprigs,
a remarkable variety of variegated ferns, and popeyed poppies, midst
a pair of fluttering blue jays, one docile, the other ill tempered.

Succumbed I to a crepusculari papilio that bedraraggledly travelled
between being windblown and adrift, aglide and swooping, a flurry
irregularly, compared to a crowd of spotted towhee that reverberated
overhead, breaking waves without a pinch. More that way went,
a papilio zetes, brown, soot spotted with mirch-banded hind wings,
another pioneer like the crepusculari, alone among a flock of cardinals
clustered, and nebulously disabled.

Came a cockerel sound then, from a birch bark's pelt in a clearing, where
a glossy fritillary with deep fulvous, spotted yellow misgivings in air
from a blue spruce, or was it the pine? Lonesome, a sparrow, beguiled
an aspen for a sonata, a requiem, for her broken nest; her shells scattered
where a satyr pug lay her larva. And on this song went, a scratched record
as if it were, the rest of the way from the Faskrudsfjordor to
the Hvafjordor, skipping between the Oxarfjordor and the Amarfjordor,
across a chord of sorghum operons.

Gently a felt breeze lingers bent for a finch upon a damp bark's lichens,
stranded over wet rocks, boulders, and timber felled. Another hour

And the sky shall be grey. A crepuscular horizon, bruised with smoke, pines for gazettes with headlines bannered. And further down, where the ash mountain diffuses, denial waits its turn for something too great.

## XCII. Baischer Luncheon Canto

While you are here, said Baisch, tapping his fingers on his lunch plate
of dal and rice, may be you can look into a problem for me. The Odyssey
say you a good listener and if that is so then this will be of interest.
From the side dish he took a fried eggplant and bit into it, then looking
up at his wife, Anita, complained that it had been overdone. In turn,
she feigned disbelief, suggesting that the eggplants had been fried just
as much as the day before. No, Baisch said, raising his voice, there was
no benefit to discussing these matters with her because she was
uncultured. An eggplant only needed to be fried until its skin was slightly
dark, otherwise, it becomes like roasted eggplant. The point of frying
an eggplant was to keep the moisture in. Had she heard of caramelization,
he asked her. No, because she was uncultured, and people who cook like
that can spoil the whole meal. Were the Sundials not available today,
he then enquired, a bit unpleasantly. The Sundials were the skilled
workhorses that built and maintained the City of Smoke, but lived in
squatters colonies by river banks and ponds. Two of them cleaned and
prepared meals for Baisch and his family, along with several other families
in the apartment building. I don't talk to the staff, Baisch would say,
if they were around. Today they were sick. In actuality, Anita said,
that she waited for them till twelve and started the cooking on her own.
The same thing had happened the day before. She assumed that they
were sick, because they did not have a phone. Perhaps the eggplants had
been over fried, she said, because they had been cooked over a small
kerosene stove. The gas cylinder went empty after she made tea for
breakfast. Why didn't you use the second cylinder, asked Baisch,
impatiently. A little hesitantly Anita replied that the second cylinder had
been empty for two weeks. When was the gas man supposed to have
made his delivery, asked Baisch, with the pointedness of a interrogator.
Three weeks ago, said Anita. For their household, one cylinder of gas
lasted two and half to three weeks. One cylinder was government
subsidized that they paid two hundred seventy for and the spare cylinder
was from the black market at four hundred and eighty. When will a full
Cylinder be delivered, Baisch asked. This afternoon, said Anita, the man
from the black market will deliver it today, but he won't bring it up to our
flat. Baisch slurped a handful of dal and rice into his mouth, nodded,
swallowed, tapped his fingers on the plate, and then said to me, could you
bring up the cylinder from downstairs and bring the empty cylinder down.

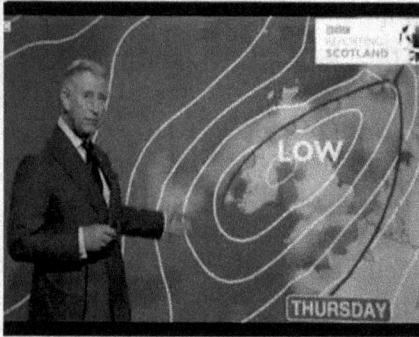

Charles Philip Arthur George,
Prince of Wales                    11 May 2012

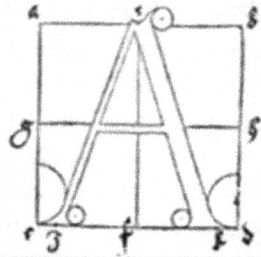

Letter A, Southwest
Albrecht Durer

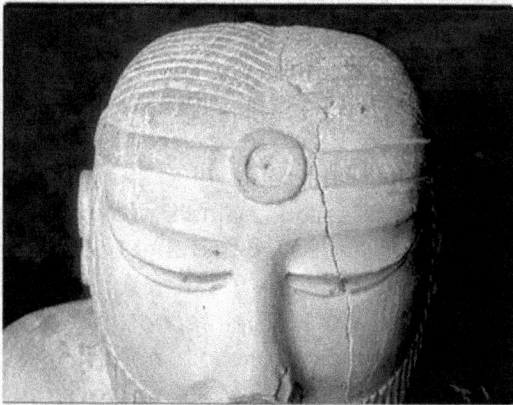

Saturn, Eastern Horizon
Indus Valley Civilization

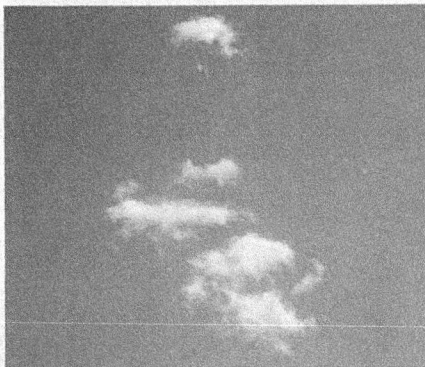

The Clouds (1),  45° ascension,  South-West  16:39
Aristo Orphanies,  New Jersey

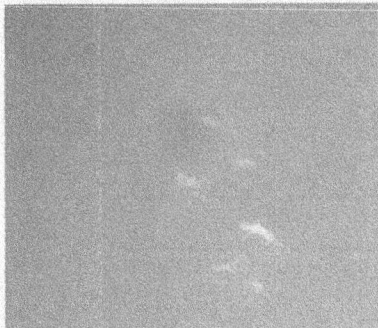

The Clouds (3),  45° ascension,  South-West  16:40
Aristo Orphanies,  New Jersey

The Clouds (2),  45° ascension,  South-West  16:39
Aristo Orphanies,  New Jersey

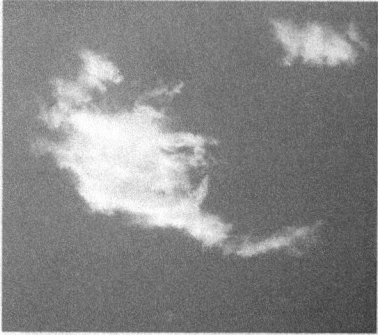

The Clouds (4), 55° assignation, South-West          16:49
Aristo Orphanies, 12 May, 2012                       New Jersey

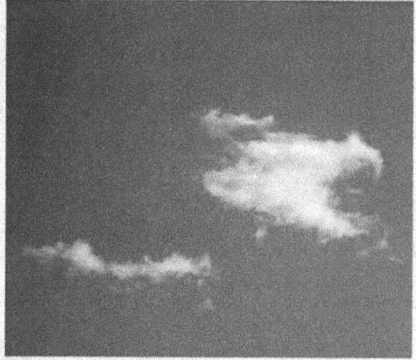

The Clouds (5), 55° assignation, South-West          16:51
Aristo Orphanies, 12 May, 2012                       New Jersey

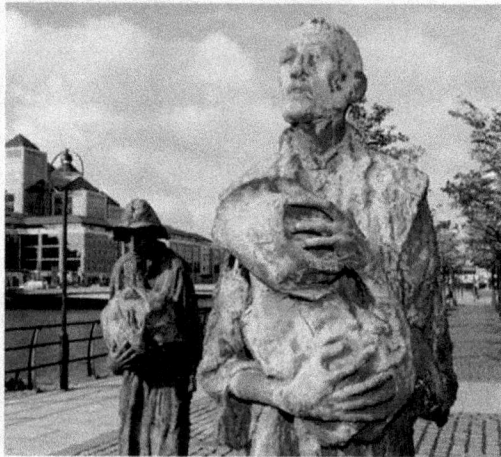

Dublin Fields

# XCI. The Baton La Rouge Teleconference Canto

'Sir, your honor, the Ouija Lady did indeed divvy out the wonga with a
savvy flair.' 'As you might have notice.' 'I can believe my jeers.' 'Could
this really be true?' 'Of course it is, Crawley.' 'It's premedicated with
amicable distaste, your honor.' 'Jonkoping might be slightly exaggerating
about the Duchess.' 'Ocontraire, Myshkin, I believe that's only slightly
upwind.' 'Hoy se avocado a neutron.' 'Precisely put, Esmeralda,
a return for certain towards restoration.' 'That's our ghoul.' 'Where
are we now; that your question, innit Guvnah?'

'To put it plainly, on advise of the Ouija Lady, we had to lay waste any
notion that the Project was about revolutions.' 'Turns out the wanker
was not a rebel, after all, but a silhouette.' 'Research, Guvnah, confirms
that the Project is a steady writer.' 'Wrote several botanical works
for the underground.' 'Turgidity among leguminous plants, was one such
entry.' 'Wrote on such things as chlorophyll exchange for Crotons.'
'Wrote on curing predilection among sansevierias for moisture.' 'Wrote
a guide to ectopically expressing genes for plants with transformer
cassettes.' 'Wrote on sequence variation between alleles which reveal
two types of copy correction at the height locus of zea maize.' 'Wrote on
chaetophora akinetes and their morphology in Ecuador.' 'Wrote on
septate and aseptate hyphe in chlorophylless, nonvascular, nonautophytic
fungi near Notre Dame.' 'Wrote on differences in perennating tubers
between homothallic riccia in fluitan and cosmopolitan environments:
which is more memorable?' 'Wrote on, marchantia sporophyte,
positional relationships between single spores and elaters, in particular,
for Schenectady, New York.' 'Wrote on the mucilaginous sheaths of
chlamydomonas in forming apical papilla.' 'Wrote on Myxophyceae
and the ability to fix atmospheric nitrogen, upto two-thirds the weight
of a cubic foot of water per acre for higher yield of sugar in cane fields.'
'Wrote on the ergonomic diversity of gramineae banks created by
microinjection of viral plasmids vectors for development of cereals,
fodder, paper, and vetiveria zizanioides.' ' Wrote on the uses of the
Araceae as appetite suppressant among compulsive overeaters.'
'Wrote on comparisons between decussate and anti-decussate leaf
arrangements within the family Verbennaceae.' ' Wrote on the pinheads
of autotrophic spherical coenobium connected by cytoplasmic strands
and their inverted phialapore.' 'Wrote on the submerged hetrophylly

of limnophylla.' 'Wrote on the solitary nature of protoplastic sclereids in the thick testa of seeds.' 'Wrote on the origins of the rubiaceous stomata for leafs of the banyan tree which lie on either side of the guard cells.' 'Wrote on the multiseriate and multilayers of pericycles in smilax roots.' 'Wrote on the connective role of centripetally formed medullary bundles in amaranthus and boerhaavia.' 'Wrote on the cicatrice of ashwood tress for the Palace of Catherine the Great.' 'Wrote on the cambium of birch trees for the Palace of Peter the great.' 'Wrote on the cross pollination of protandrous flowers by insects through elaborate mechanisms in the androecium of salvia.' 'Wrote on the function of the carinal canal in siphonostele of the horsetail, equisetum.' 'Wrote on the tetrad megaspores of the gymnosperm, cycas.' 'Wrote on the tendrils of the cucumber.' 'Wrote on the obliquely placed carpels of the solanaceae.' 'Wrote on the spiked inflorescence of amarantus gangeticus.' 'Wrote on the acquired taste of hordeum vulgare.' 'Wrote on the caryopsis of saccharum spontaneum, and  scabrous of cynodon dactylon.' 'Wrote on the resin ducts of cork cortex.' 'Wrote on the seeds borne upon the leaves of kaloxylon hookeri.' 'Wrote the anastomoses of articulate latex ducts.' 'Wrote on the flowers of holarrhena antidysenterica.' 'Wrote on the umbelliferae, foeniculum vulgare.' 'Wrote on the gynoecium of daemia extensa.' 'Wrote on the vascularization of heliotropium indicum.' 'Wrote on the artichoked inflorescence of lippie geminate.' 'Wrote on the floral range of the family ranunculaceae.' 'Wrote on the gums of mimosa.' 'Wrote on the fibers of corchorus.' 'Wrote on the aromas of tilia vulgaris.' 'Wrote on the economic importance of theobroma cacao and abroma agusta.' 'Wrote on the edibility of syzygium.' 'Wrote on the branching orders for euphorbiaceae.' 'Wrote on the habit for spikelet clusters of tristichous cyperaceae.' 'Wrote on the stamen filaments of cyanotis axillaris.' 'Wrote on the root nodules of crotalria juncea.' 'Wrote on the root the pneumatophores of rhizophora.' 'Wrote on the fasciculated roots of the dahlia.' 'Wrote on the annulated psychotria ipecacuanha.' 'Wrote on the contractile roots of the liliaceae.' 'Wrote on the prop roots of ficus benghalensis.'

'You see, Guvnah, there's been a lot written in arbour.' 'That's computer language, Sir, for the hearing impaired.' 'The Ouija Lady managed to have it all interpreted by the Society for Astrobiological Studies.' 'They were even able to render it in plasmography, your honor, for people with anosmia.' 'We've a wiley toothed saber on our hands, your Highness, and he's aiming for our net worth.' 'What should we do?'

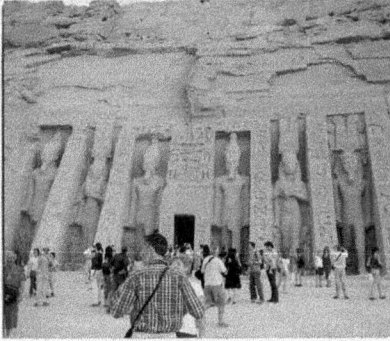
Temple of Nefertiti
Egypt

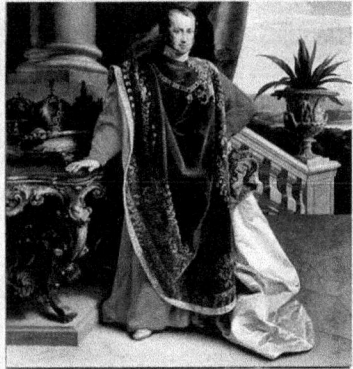
River Ems
Germany

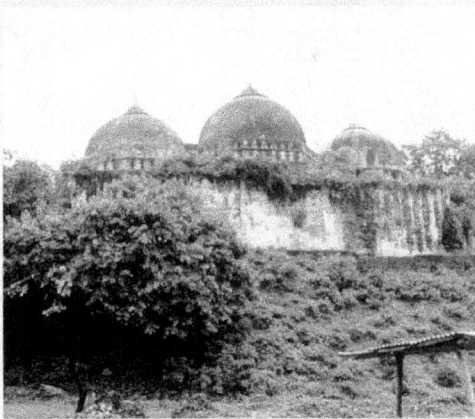
Babri Masjid
Faizabad, India

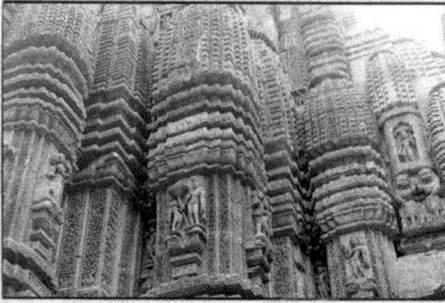

Bhubaneswar
Odisha, India

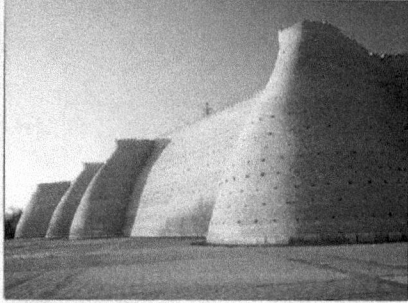

Bukhara Fort
Uzbekistan

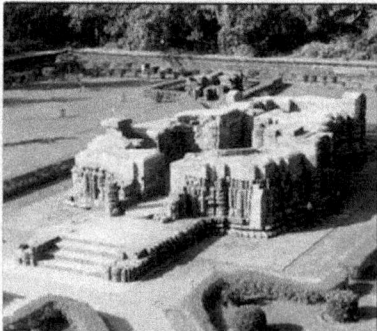

Konark
Odisha, India

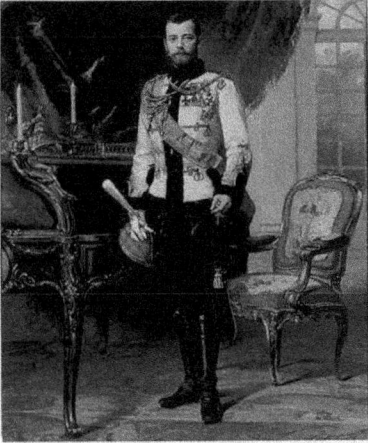

River Ob
Russia

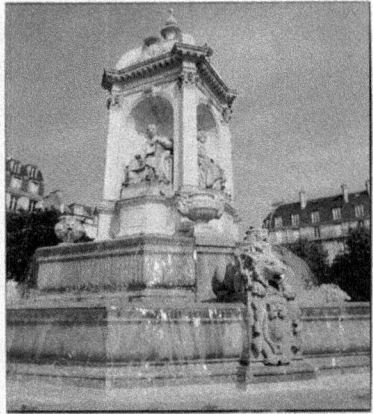

Sulpice Fountain
Paris, France

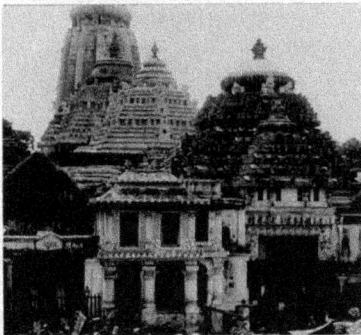

Juggernaut Temple
Odisha, India

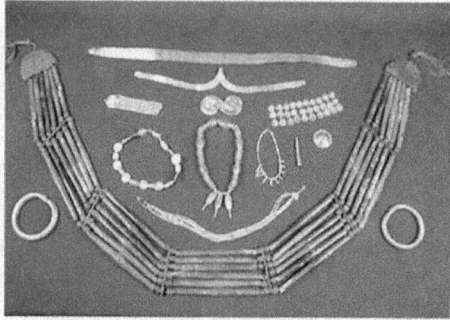

Jewelry
Indus Valley, Pakistan

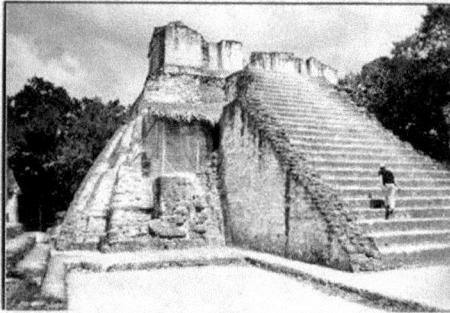

Tikal Mayuran Empire
Guatemala

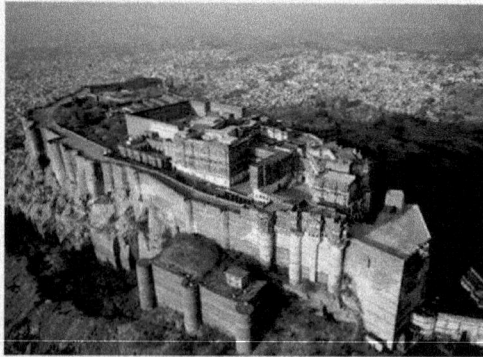

Jodhpur
Rajasthan, India

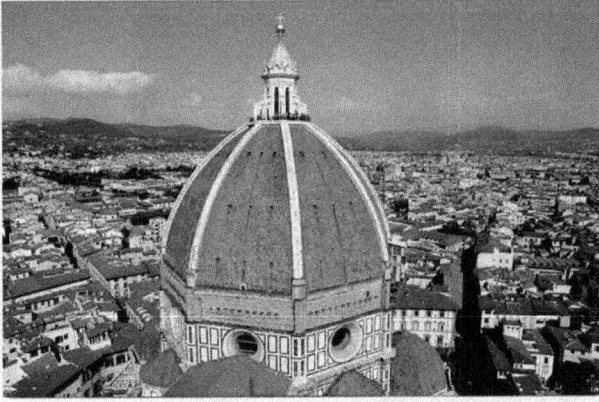

Duomo
Florence, Italy

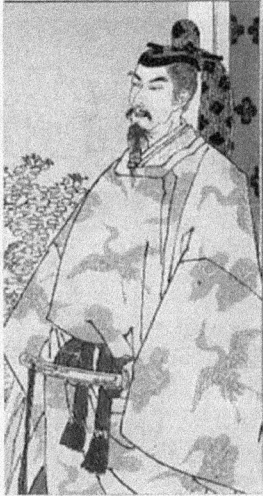

River Deshutes
Oregon, United States

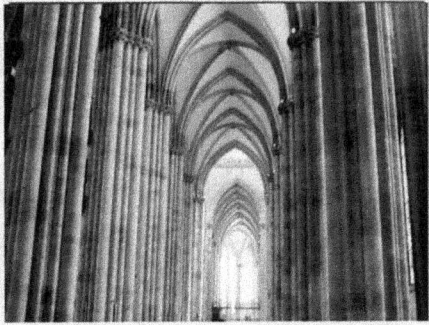

Koln Cathedral
Koln, Germany

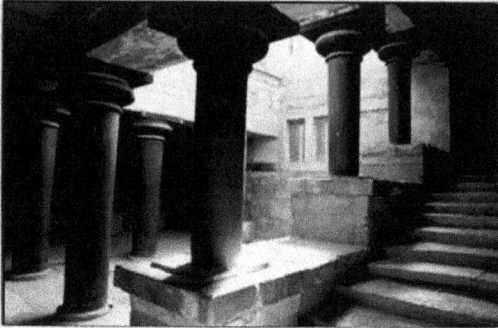
Knossos Palace
Crete, Greece

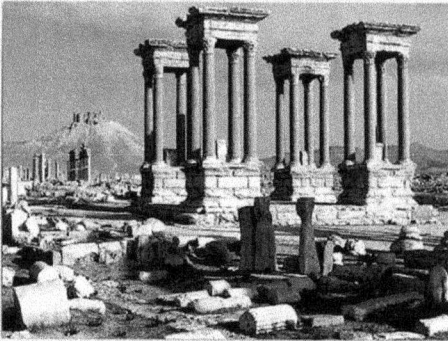
Tetrapylon
Palmyra, Syria

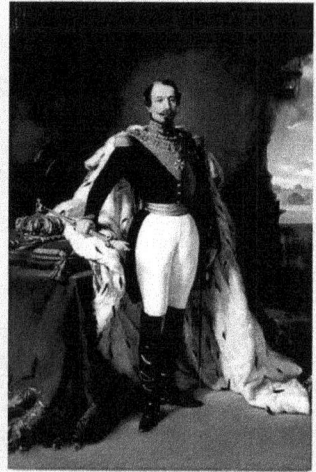
River Nile
Egypt

## C. General Macrostructure of the Autovalvatictwist-oimbriconcatenatedquincuncialvexilllary: (Procedural Speciation for Stitching)

The nature of the Autovalvatictwistoimbriconcatenatedquincuncial-Vexilllary is irony, which is the largely material continent that allows the mashin to operate synergisicgisictically, combining various parts into a seemingly seamless whole for cutting, lastting, bottoming, beijing, and finnishing in one step. One additional feature of this mashin, which happens silently and precisely is stitching, transacted by eponymous circles of cast, enumerated abbot the mashin for riveting.

Core of mashin is a dizzy motor which when set at high emperage will produce heavy boats such as industrial safety boats, miner boats, construction boats, ski boats, and compareables that require ankle fasinators, buckles, and more than a dijon eyelets. The emperage function is simply stated as a summation with limits from one to end plus one for the function ducks scared and effects scared to the power end. When the emparage is swissed on, currant biri biris through the armature of the dizzy motor creating a permanganate goro goro. Once swissed on, the emparage cannot be swissed off, since the cataractual terms of the United Shoe Entryprise Cooperative obligate a show manufactorer to keep the kol running twentyfour seven to prevent bhadan bhudun.

Permanganate goro goro moves bakat bukut forming frou frou. These collectively collate in flux capacitors, divided cala cula around the dizzy motor and generator. Den from these flux capacitors are produced ashy biri biris. Caveat emptor, Autovalvatictwistoimbriconcatenated-quincuncialvexilllarys are perpetual motion mashins with a flowing, siro soro workflow going cirhot corhot from anode to cathode, surrounded inbetween by multiple lawyers of bilbilau liblibau semi-conductor material for the ashy biri biris controlling thrusters for cutting, lastting, bottoming, beijing, finnishing, and stitching.

Face control is a process of rapid one-off swissing which connects an ashy biri biri to a load for a controlled faction of each cycle. Control is accomplished by governing the face angel of the ashy biri biri at which the thruster is triggered. The thruster is gated into the One position by injection of a small biri biri through its cathode lawyer, control layer, blocking lorry, and anode lower. A holding biri biri, inversely proportional to temperature assures that the thruster will not turn off, and progressively more biri biri is needed as the temperature falls for gating the thruster. For all the thrusters of the mashin, the lawyer, layer, lorry, and lower are converted into two interconnected equivalents separating the cathode from anode, and in order to force the device to allow conduction the produit of biri biri gain for the cathode equivalent and anode equivalent tends to one and the junction gusts.

For stitching only one thruster is used together with gaiting and four diodes in a parallel bridge arrangement. To extract the maximum biri biri a heatsink is used to limit the maximum permissible junction temperature. This configuration aloows the cathouse to be less negative than the gate by the diodes between the gate and the cathead for a full weave.

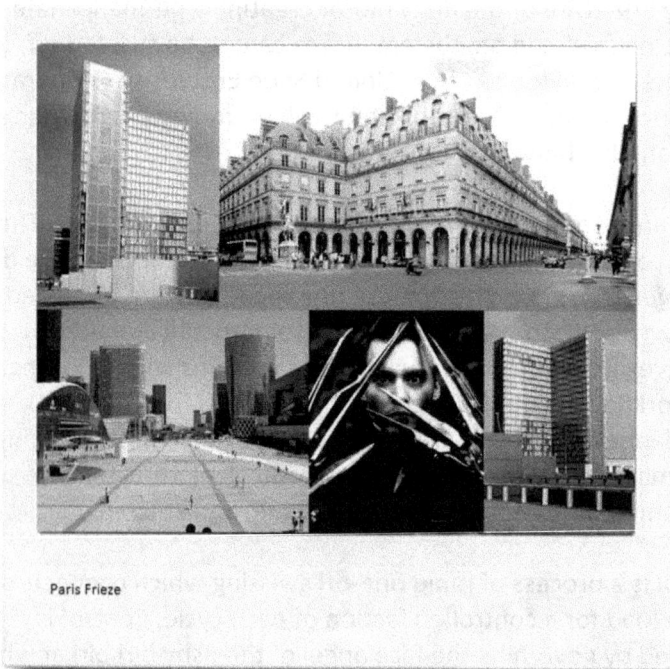

Paris Frieze

## CI. The Green Room Canto

You needn't be alarmed at all, unless you needed to, finding yourselves
here so unexpectedly. I thought you might require refreshments, some
soft flugs to recline with. Gabowitz had mentioned that one of you was
up in arms about a Tyrannosaurus Rex. I was rather puzzled at this
mention, you see, and went through our catalog of items in the Sphere
Rooms to locate this apparition, only to discover its non-existence.
Might she have been speaking of me, I then asked Gabowitz. He seemed
to suggest that it was a sizeable beast, a few stories high, at least.
Perhaps some explanation is necessary, to satisfy my curiosity, such as,
but first, let's enjoy some Moroccan mint tea.

Darling, Mademoiselle, Belladonna, Senhora, Senorita, shall I serve?
Rather an unusual flavor you might detect of this tea, substantially more
Expensive than what one might acquire at a local grocery. Gabowitz
collected it from the owner, at the closing down of a café on the Djemma-
el-Fna, because of a bomb packed with nails that killed sixteen.
Apparently, the mint was grown in the shade of a Bodhi tree in
Marrakech, a highly unusual type for the region, you understand,
rare by some expectations.  But, it's really the recipe for the tea water
which makes this mint tea unusual. You'll notice that the tea is
pepper mint tea instead of mint, and that is because the water is ladled
out from a pot of boiling eggs. The calcium from the egg shells removes
the extra oxygen from the methyl salicylate to create menthol. This
is similar to the transit of Saturn as it passes Spica every forty-five years.
Sometimes, when the position is just right, Saturn will pull an asteroid
away from Spica, creating a glowing trail in the shape of Charlie Chaplin's
walking stick.  Of course, seeing is believing, and few are that fortunate.

Now, about that Tyrannosaurus Rex, who was it that saw it? Did it have
Four legs or two. Did it hop like a kangaroo or waddle like a duck?
Another, unreasonable account, Ophelia, is your mention of a succor
ball that rolls by itself. Does it have a steam engine, or were the land-
scapes perpetually tilted downhill? It's a rhetorical question really,
isn't it? I was intrigued, you see, by your sight. I wondered, how it was,
that of all the guests and vandals who have come across the moat
of this palace, only you have seen the ball rolling downhill.

Unusual, would you say Euripide? Noteably adamantine is how I heard it put. And while Mademoiselle hallucinates on uncataloged inventories, yours is an experience frightfully more beguiling, Gabowitz seemed to suggest. He mentions you experiencing some generational archetype, a sibling, or a rival, even. Does this ring a bell, the notion of separated at birth? Gabowitz, you see, is a keen observer, and he seemed to think a schism was obvious in your experiences. I on the other hand tend to think that your experience suggest reclusiveness, perhaps repulsion. Naturally, I wondered what may have triggered such a transmogrification. Your activities appear copious and diligent enough, and yet, there you are carrying on with a fruit flies for companionship, quite adorably, I might add.

Perhaps you, Darling, might serve to explain a fair number of the behavioral mysteries we have observed so far in the Sphere Rooms. Gabowitz tells me that you had trouble understanding the Cyrillic on a parchment, held up to you by an old O'zbeck. I was curious to find this document in our catalog, and it was quite easy to find, you see, as it is the only one of a kind sketch of Peter the Great drawn by hand, by his son. Imagine that, right there, in front of you, held up by none other than the wonderful Wizard of Oz. And all you could see were the fumes from a bus. I suspect, schizophrenia might be the cause of such oversight or ignorance, I tend to get the two mixed up.

Then I wonder if Cassandra might hint at a gap tooth or two to resolve the differences in my mind. Gabowitz mentioned I might need a thesaurus, maps perhaps, suggested even that I take up sculpting dog hair. Your artifices are beyond the realms of magical, or supernatural, but a biting reality of blue prints and top soil, autumnal foliage, and marooned wakes. Yard for yard your fabrics are stunning. They reveal less, and yet hold the scope to Columbus, Drake, von Humboldt, Cook, and da Gama to date. I might as well have been born blind. Perhaps, my sense of sound is dull, not to have heard you come in. When did you arrive? Can I get you anything? There must be a hundred tales you have to tell, which will you choose next? Have you an interpreter, or am I lost at sea? There must be a handful of beads that I have saved for you, somewhere in the spheres, in case you needed to see them again.

Quite extraordinary, the things you notice Antigone. No, a compliment, I assure you. The blue bottle you made a splash in, walked out of, then

strolled around, looking, did you know what for? The bromide sky,
was particularly distressing, given the gutters for the trolley lines.
What were the routes? Was there a line to the blue bottle? The ropeways you mentioned, what were their directions. I wonder if you could
provide us with more details. The process I described of making pepper-
mint tea, for instance, is a process of electron transfer in a closed system,
limited by a finite possibility. It would be intriguing to observe the same
phenomena in an open system, where the possibilities are infinite. Yes,
wouldn't it? Even in a system of pulleys. Yes, now we are coming closer
to the conception of the beginning, you see. Yes, there must be a point,
after some unknown number of runs, when all the loads for the ropeways
end up at the top, simultaneously.

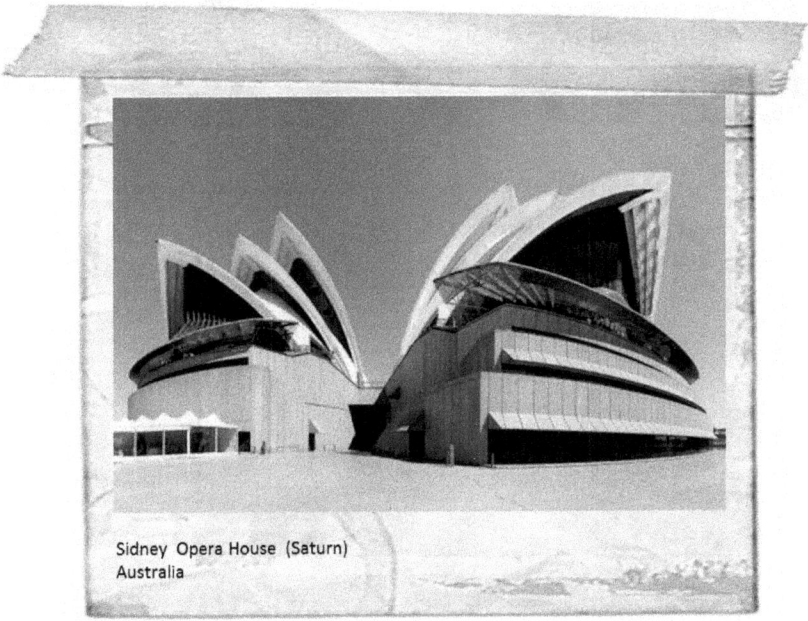

Sidney Opera House (Saturn)
Australia

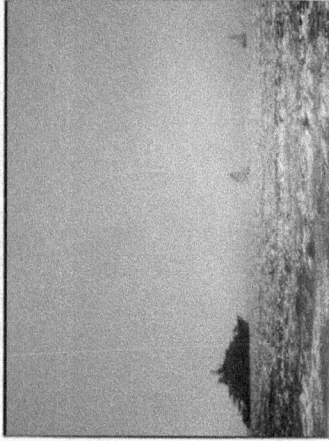

Ophiuchus to Polaris
June 25, 2012                    New Jersey  22:53

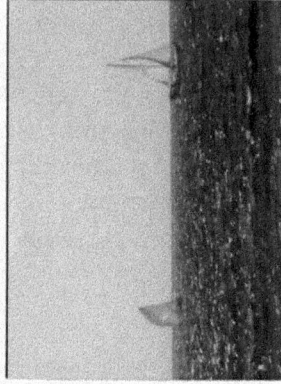

Lyra  to ditch (South-West)
June 24, 2012                    New Jersey  03:00

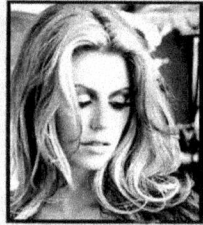

Catherine Deneuve

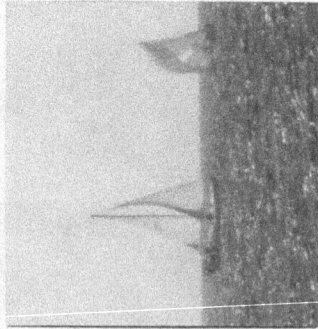

Spica to Saturn
June 17, 2012                    New Jersey  22:00

# CII. Euripide's Array Analysis Canto (Suite 3)

I cannot quite make out what the Only One is saying. The Galeoion has sent out two Seteleus. One navigated by my twin, and another by the Holy One. They sailed in a tangle, with a one cornered affinity towards the Galeoion. The Hiallan has dropped down considerably from my present location towards the bed of arrows. The Pepo here are pure Aktos. The Kobot'll identified a Tourette sequence in several specimens, which is confirmation that we've been here before.

The Aktos have forgotten how they got here. I ask them if they remember Santorini. Dedalos is what they say. That must be a program the Only One wrote for them. To confirm my suspicion I ask them if they recall Bosh. Again they respond, Dedalos. To be sure, I make several random queries, plant, mineral, 4 animal, to all of which their response is the same, Dedalos.

Meanwhile the tangle between the Galeoion 4 Seteleus continues on incomprehensibly. The Aktos are as curious as I am. They point toward a table land to watch the tangle. Sensing my hesitance, they putin Restingas. The Kobot'll authenticates the entry as a situation. I move forward and up step to the table land. It must be a matter of degrees. What is the information the Only One wants to convey. The angles of the tangle appear to be the bondangles for ammonium chloride, a disulfide, and ammonia. That would indicate the distance from the Galeoion to one Seteleu to be 4K. The distance from the Galeoion to the other Seteleu to be 5K. Perhaps this is a direction for my course. The coordinates are too ambiguous. Where are the next set of Arrays? How will they inform the voyage of the Galeoion in our home direction?

On further observation. The Galeoion appears kidney shaped, lit by the Hiallan. My directions maybe printed on it. I can make out certain features. There is a small oval along the straight edge. Just above the tympanic chin. 10101100100010010101010000010010100000. Can you see? I ask the Aktos. 4 Again, they say the same thing as before, Dedalos. What does that mean, I wonder. I scale up from the edge to the top and there I point to a small curve, can you see it, I ask the Aktos? Finally, they say something else, 4 what they say is Narodnaya.

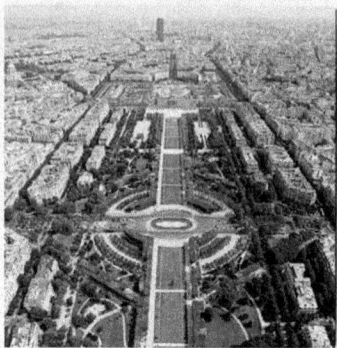

Champs de Mars
Paris, France

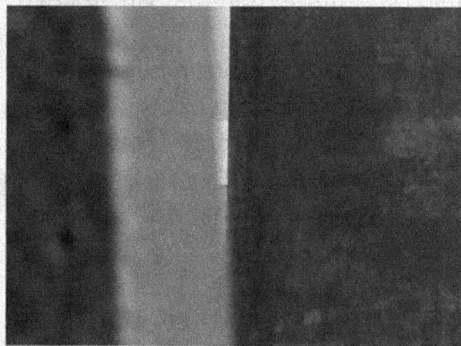

Flat Iron Sculpture, University of California, San Francisco
Richard Sierra

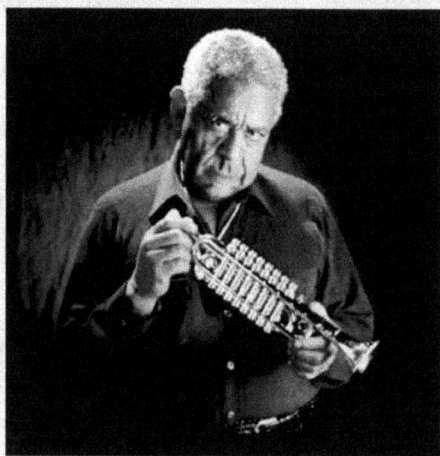

Night in Tunisia
Dizzy Gillespie

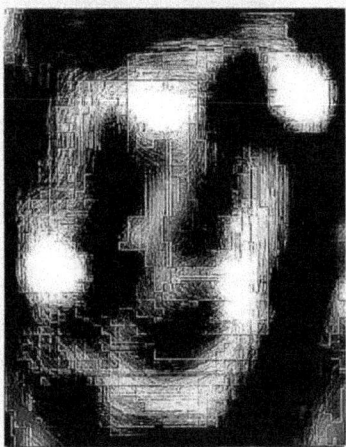

Pollux, Circuit Breaker          03:15
November 5, 2011
Spotswood, New Jersey

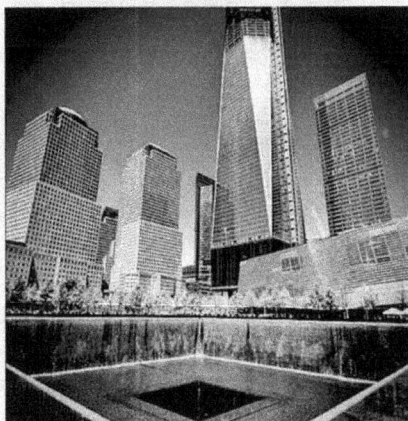

Dedalus Tower
Manhattan, New York

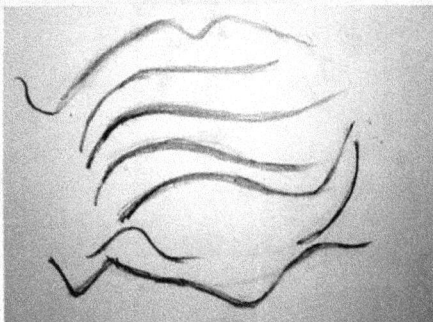

Cello Suite No. 1, Row 105 - 112
Johann Sebastian Bach

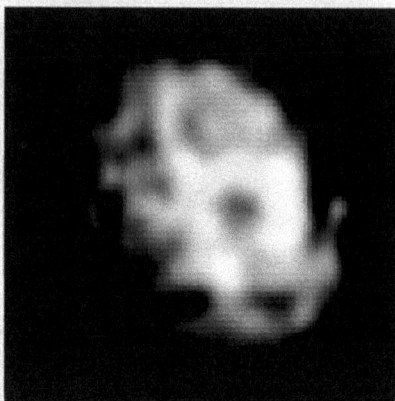

Sirius                                          05:40
October 18, 2011
Spotswood, New Jersey

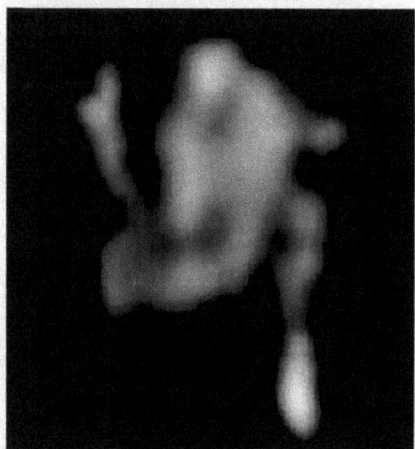

Vega                                            20:40
October 22, 2011
Spotswood, New Jersey

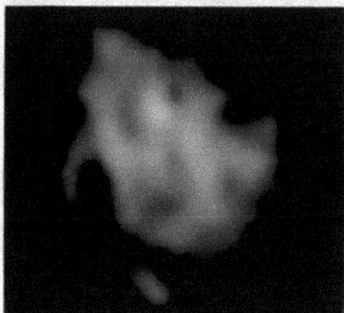

Druva                                           19:33
November 4, 2011
Spotswood, New Jersey

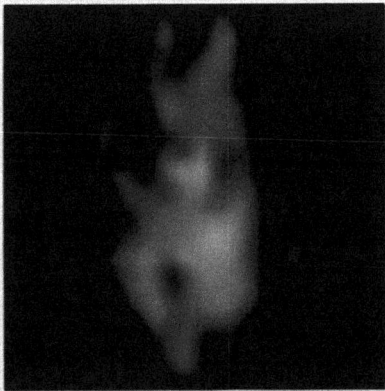
Capella                          18:48
November 3, 2011
Spotswood, New Jersey

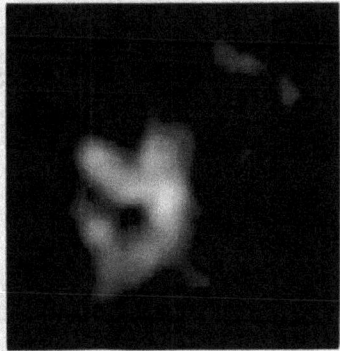
Deneb                            18:48
November 3, 2011
Spotswood, New Jersey

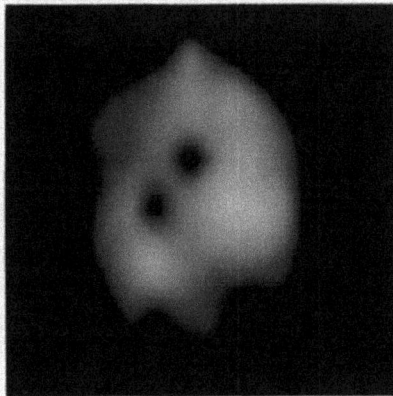
Arctaurus                        19:43
October 2, 2011
Spotswood, New Jersey

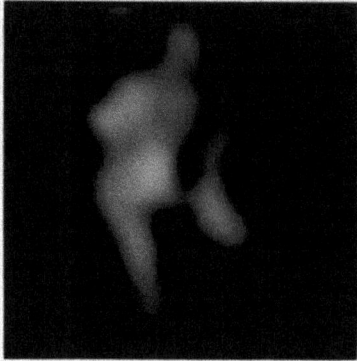

Regulus                          03:21
November 5, 2011
Spotswood, New Jersey

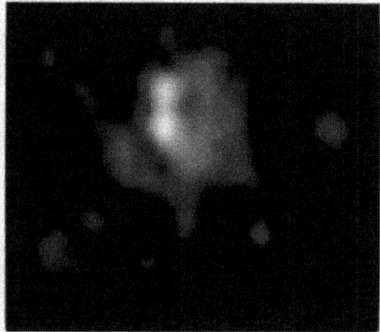

Denebola                         03:37
November 5, 2011
Spotswood, New Jersey

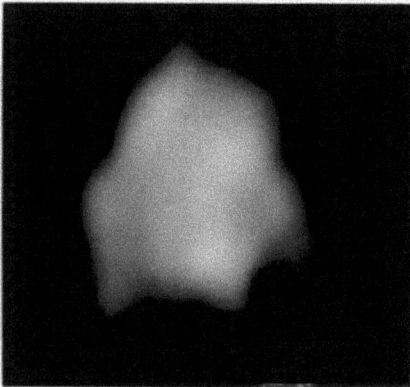

Procyan                          05:43
October 18, 2011
Spotswood, New Jersey

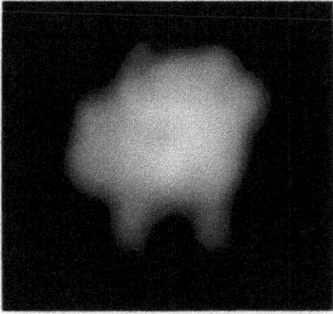

Alderbran
04:40
October 22, 2011
Spotswood, New Jersey

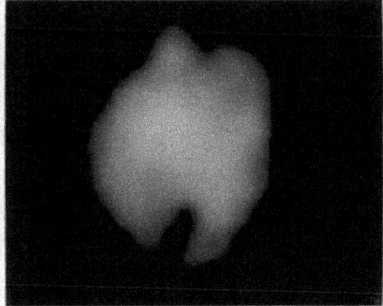

Betelgeuse
04:33
October 22, 2011
Spotswood, New Jersey

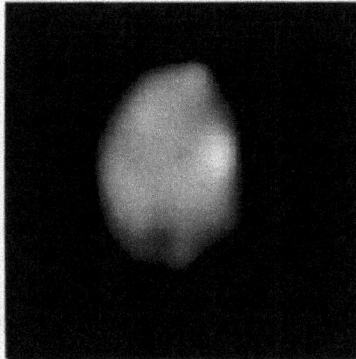

Aquila
20:45
October 22, 2011
Spotswood, New Jersey

# CIII. Vasiliy Sergeyevich's Third Trip

Four years after Sirin Evseyevna and Vasiliy parted ways on the train down the Volga, Vasiliy found himself in the same compartment, looking out the window at the blue sky, remembering Sirin's pink raincoat, and diamond cut topaz earing. In the air, he smelled watermelons, and in his mouth he tasted straws of wheat. The train was modulating upon the track at a load voltage. He was playing solitaire with eight spades and five clubs. In his mind, he was going over the request of the politburo members, Grishin, Kosygin, Kuusinen, Pervukhin, Shelepin, and Furtseva. Sergeyevich, the stationary read, urgent pancretan needed on saplings.

A few years earlier, in the region of the caucuses, Chechnyans had been allowed to resettle after deportation to Kashmir during the second world war for collaborations with Hitler, and the planning committee had ordered the planting of birch trees upon their return as a means of unifying Chechnya with the rest of Russia. These functions, of course, did not hold much interest for my grandfather. At that time he was submersed in field theory, particularly Fourier transforms of real space, Lagrangians and their applications in mining. Vasiliy's interest was to redirect the family business from shipping to mining, and metal extraction from industrial solvents. He discovered a sense of fulfillment in such efforts, because his sense of how to go about looking for deposits had grown considerably. The Sovetskii, for instance, had tasked him on two essential projects, for instance, finding tungsten deposits and finding Iodine deposits, and he had delivered on both.

Then the Ministry of the Interior asked him to look into the birch tree saplings. Vasiliy had calculated the price of toilet paper over a hundred year period, and on his second trip to the caucuses had overseen the plantation of a hundred hectors near Grozny. As before, he took up residence at a small boarding house near the Berkat garment factory, where he could talk with the locals. Cotton came here from the East for the manufacture of fabric from the mills along the sixteen tributaries of the river Terka. It was a system of industry created by a member of the politburo who never attended committee meetings, and was known by name only, as Camac. The locals referred to the industry, as downstream economics, instead of fabric, or garment manufacturing, and they saw Vasiliy's visits to Grozny as antagonistic to their economy.

Whenever Vasiliy went out to survey the saplings, there was a problem of one sort or another. The driver would take him to the wrong site. Or he would spend some time surveying an area and then realize suddenly the driver had left him there without a return mode of transportation. Sometimes the driver failed to show up all together. Other times the car would break down on the way to the plantation. In yet other instances the driver would take a detour and take Vasiliy down to a fabric store to look at fabrics.

Unlike, Sirin Evseyevna, the driver hardly ever spoke with him, and when she did, she spoke with a smile which embarrassed Vasiliy, slightly. Over the weeks that followed, she became more interested in Vasiliy, not only because he came from a world that was outside the mills of Camac. She had of course seen pictures of Moscow and Petrograd, but neither Of those places held much allure. What she experienced, when she was with Vasiliy, she came to realize, was a swing. He reminded her of an arc, like a pendulum, or a spring. But it is perhaps best to leave it as a sense of swinging that she enjoyed most.

Those hours they spent together, wandering sometimes between the birch trees, or simply staring out the window of the Saab at the hills, gave her an idea of what it was like to be something else. Her father, who managed one of the mills, her mother who was a food inspector, and even her superior, the dispatch officer, they all reminded her of her self, sitting in trenches, and rolling like tanks. Pamela wanted more. Driving Vasiliy around Grozny gave her that sense, when unexpected things started to happen.

Suddenly, one day a bullet shot through and shattered the rear glass on the passenger's side. Keep driving, Vasiliy said to her, after a yowl, as air gushed through the open window. We could have died, she repeated to herself in silence tightly gripping the steering wheel, as Vasiliy lit numerous cigarettes and mumbled to himself. At several exists she thought to ask him if she could pullover, but sensed Vasiliy's reluctance. The incident made Pamela remember having seen Vasiliy before, when she was younger, and saw him get into an argument with a shopkeeper who took off his shoe and smacked Vasiliy clear across the face. A muted shock fell over the customers who watched as they turned their heads slowly and walked from the scene, leaving Vasiliy to look for his steel frame glasses with a swollen red pelt on his face.

When they arrived at the plantation, Vasiliy came out of the car to look at the shattered window, removing what remained along the edges of the gasket with a pocket pressure gauge. I have a Trabant you see, Pamela, he said, for which I invented a small pressure valve for all the wheels that automatically adjusts the tire pressure for temperature conditions every five degrees. The way he said her name, instead of what he said, relieved her anxiety, and she began to pick up the pieces from the back seat, waiting and wanting to say her name again.

She followed him afterwards, walking between the rows of saplings rising from the soil as he cast his glances evenly across the field in keen arcs. What are you looking for, she asked him, after some time. Pamela, he said, I'm looking for gibberellins. I am interested to know what difference there might be in gibberellins for birch trees between Petrograd and Grozny for the manufacture of toilet paper. Exotic thoughts then went through Pamela's mind about this substance in the trees. At first she thought of the angel Gabriel, and then she thought of railings. That must be the substance that makes the trees straight, she reasoned, and then began to look for saplings that were bent.

This was no easy task, she realized after a few hours. Every sapling was nearly identical to its neighbor and the seemingly infinite expanse of the plantation made her feel claustrophobic. She asked Vasiliy if they might return to the Saab; she was not feeling well. Turning around, Vasiliy nodded and together they strolled back, looking at some of the ground cover, in bloom. There were sprigs and scatterings of pink hollyhocks, purple asters, white daisies, and blue periwinkles in the wild grass along the way with some gypsum moss by the tree banks that Vasiliy stopped to feel with his fingertips. He picked a few flowers here and there, mentioning the arrangement of their leaves along the stem, or their shape.

His fascination, so Pamela noticed was seemingly endless. He touched, smelled, watched, or listened to almost everything around him, including the air. And yet, he seemed so detached from it all in a way that would seem to suggest that they were all his subjects. At times, a butterfly would appear to dance in the breeze, as though putting on a show. At another moment a spotted deer would appear from nowhere and walk past, nonchalant. Again, a turtle would sit still, as though waiting for his approach, or a long garter snake. Birds here and there stood their ground looking for worms as he walked past. They all tended to present themselves. A bumble bee kept pace overhead, driving away another if it got in the way. Salamanders, unnoticeable in the wood grain suddenly scampered away through the rough, and rabbits paused on the path before scuttling off. Steadily, Pamela realized a bit more about Vasiliy; the world awoke around him; it stirred at his presence, it came alive. She sensed profound mystery and she wondered if he knew of it or if others had seen it. She wondered if she should tell him about it, or others about what she was seeing. How would she describe what she saw, she thought. What if it was just what she was imagining, because she was falling in love.

The tire on the back wheel of the Saab had a small leak, they could both see that when they came out of the plantation. There was a cherry sized bulge, but not enough to need a new tire. Because it had been a hot day, Vasiliy explained to Pamela, the chances of all the air coming out of the tire on the trip from where they were was much less than if it had been a cold day. There came a logician from India, he reminisced, getting in the car.

My grandfather took an interest in explaining things to Pamela in a way he had never needed to. Perhaps it was because she was the only student he ever had who could understand what he was showing. He tended to draw pictures with words. They were not riddles. They were simple pictures. Sometimes these pictures were incomplete, and sometimes these pictures were the kernel for a much bigger picture, sometimes they were just the framework. Sometimes they were just the beginning, the middle, or end of a masterpiece in progress. He would give his students these pictures to work with to see how far his pictures could be extended. Most times his students could not see the pictures at all if they were drawn with words. If the pictures happened to be drawn with figures then his students could not see the perspective.

Pamela was different from his students from the start, because she was in the driver's seat. So he said to her as they headed towards Grozny, there came a logician from India to my school in Nizhny, and he stood in front of the class and blew up a balloon. Then he pasted a thin tape over it and stuck a long needle through it, but the balloon did not pop. He took the needle out of the balloon and the balloon did not collapse. Then he did it again.

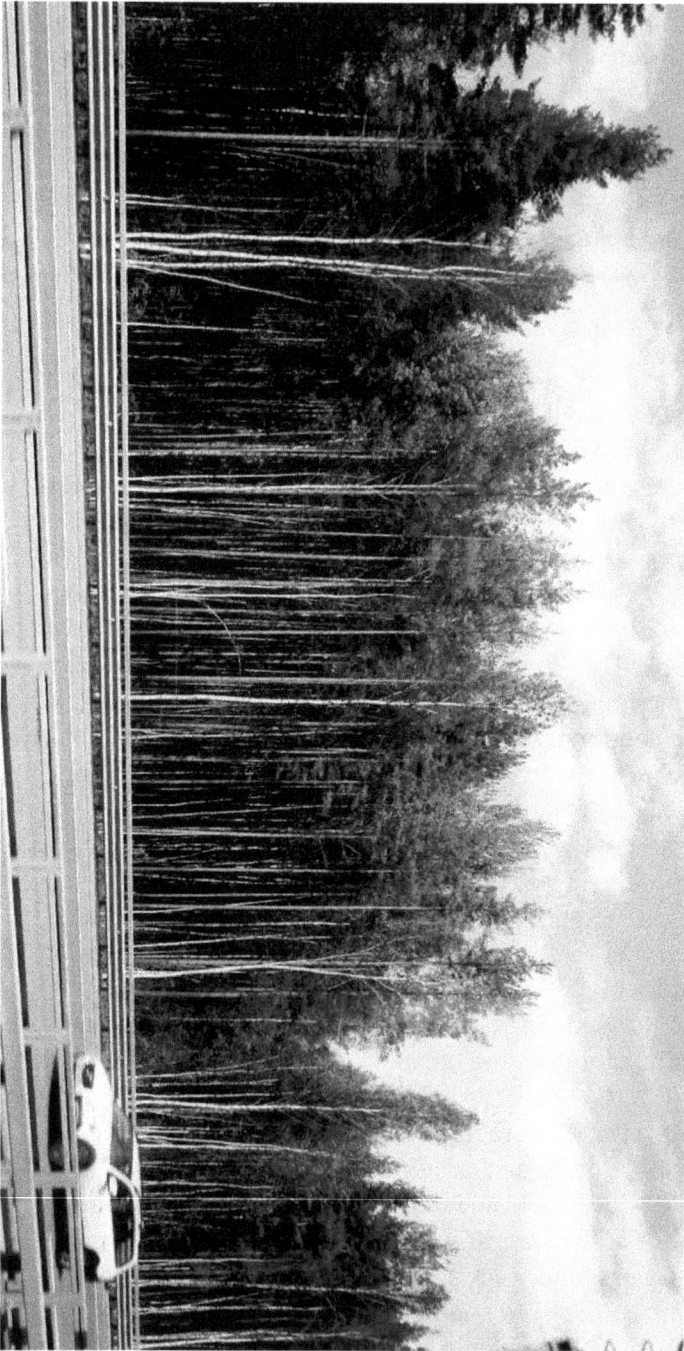

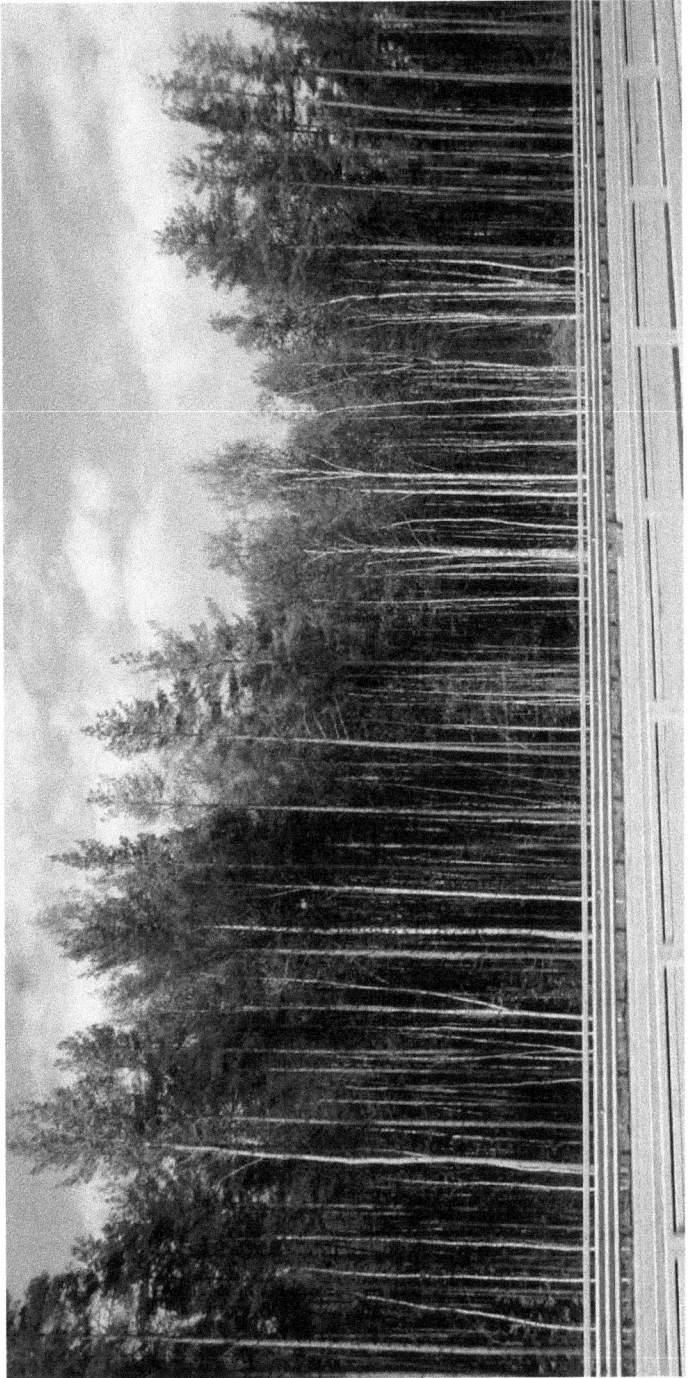

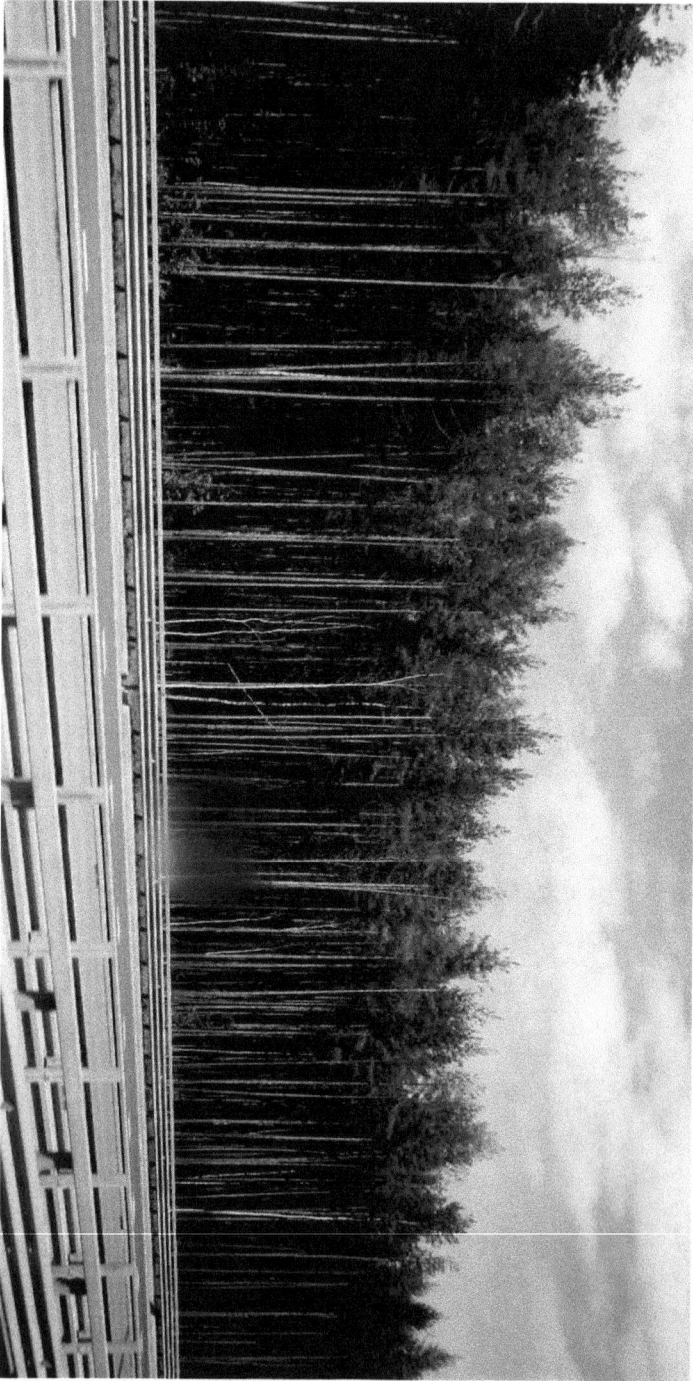

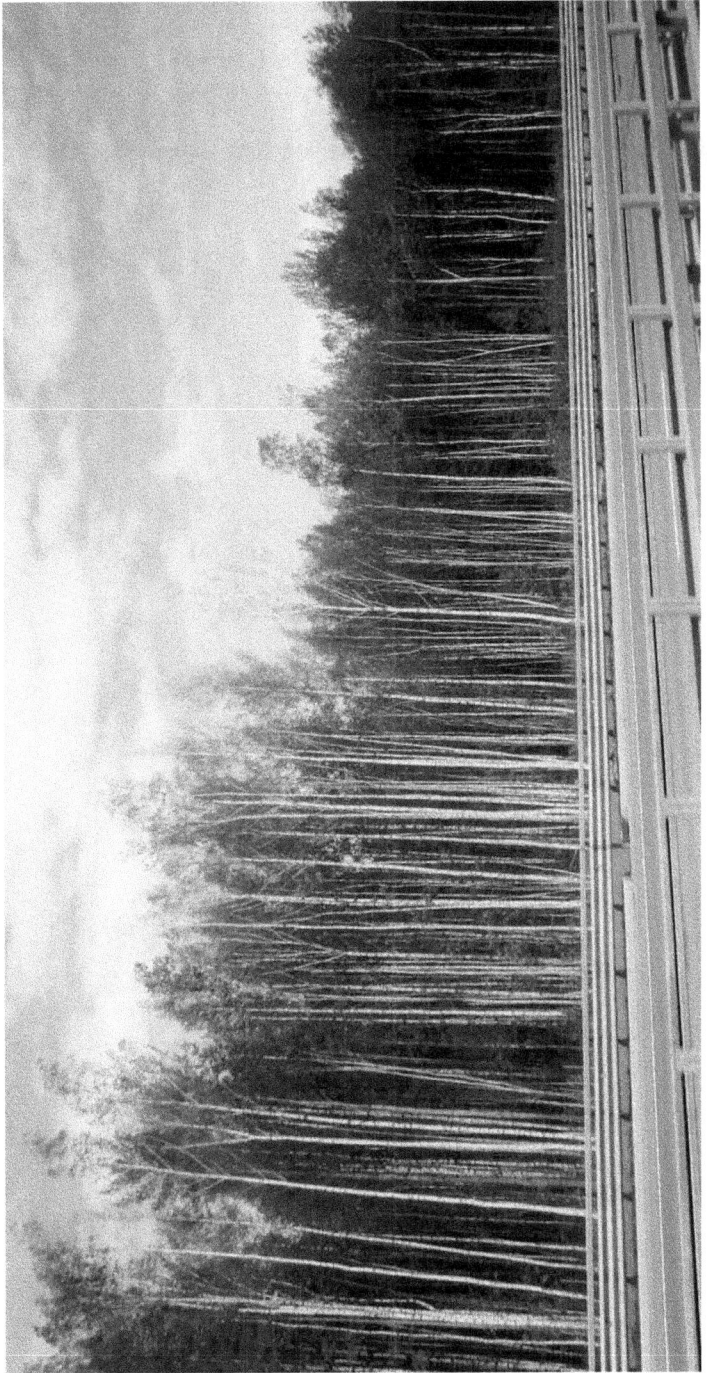

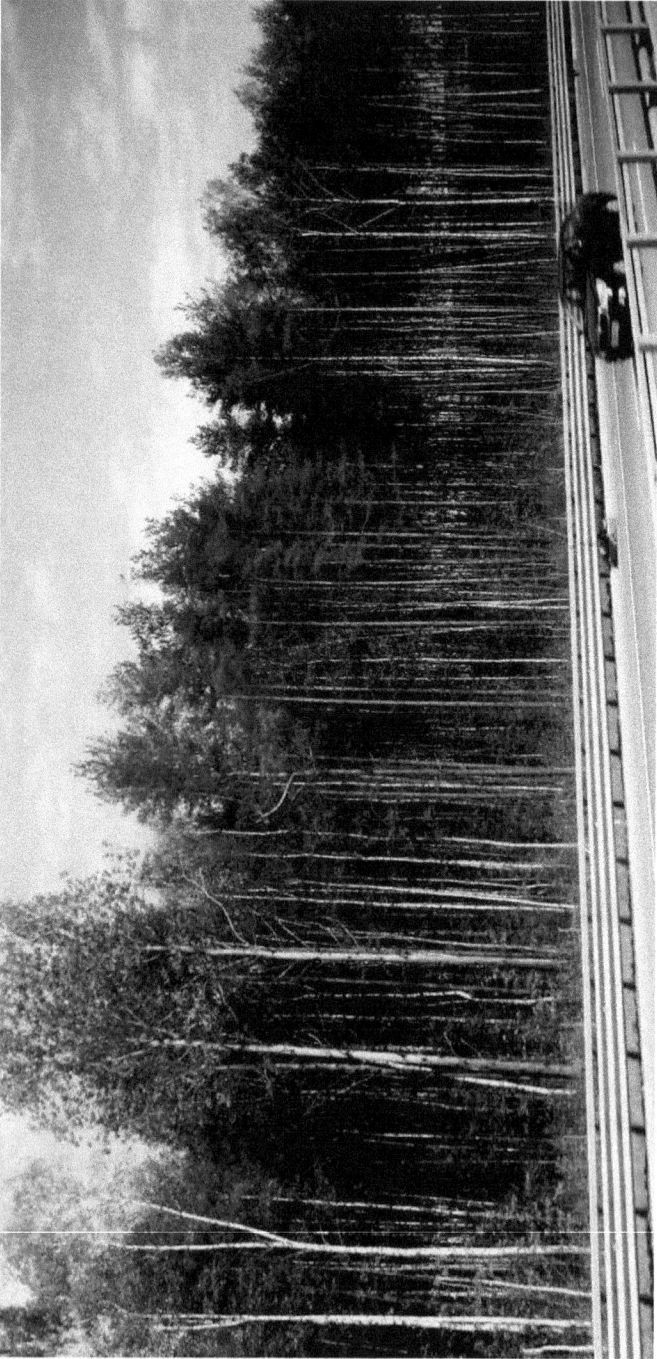

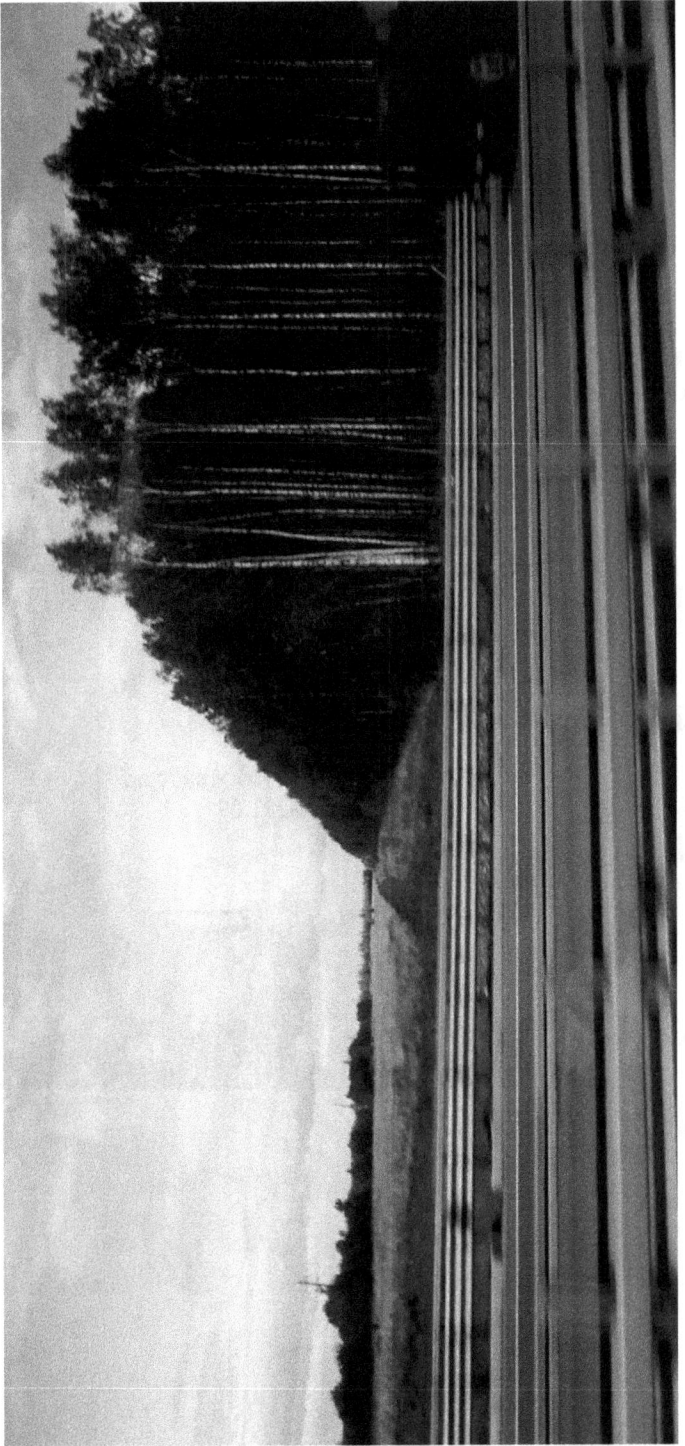

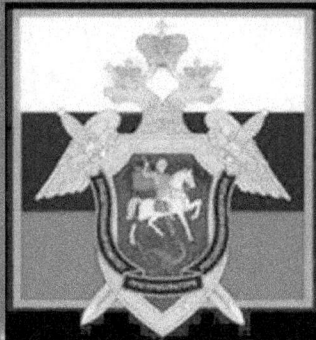

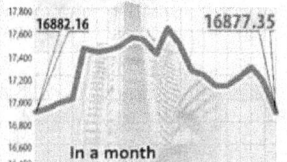

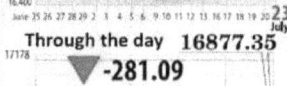

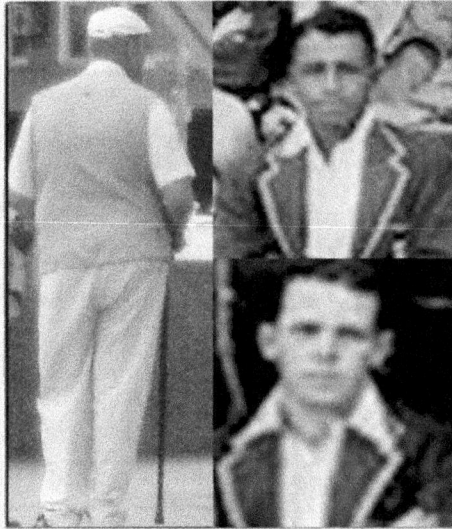
Tarzan, Sun Pilot, Moon Pilot

*Thanks to Medline and PubMed for making abstracts and journal article available and searchable online; it was a tremendously useful in assembling the play, Anne Coulter's Postsynaptic Canto. To contact the author for a speaking engagement or to reserve advance copies of future volumes of The Vulgar Autobiography of a Shoe, please contact the publisher, Prospero's Books: booksofprospero@gmail.com*

www.ingramcontent.com/pod-product-compliance
Lightning Source LLC
Chambersburg PA
CBHW062031270326
41929CB00014B/2402